Ultrasound Diagnosis of Breast Diseases

For Churchill Livingstone

Publisher: Geoff Nuttall
Senior Project Controller: Neil A. Dickson
Project Controller: Nicky S. Carrodus
Indexer: Nina Boyd
Sales Promotion Executive: Douglas McNaughton

Ultrasound Diagnosis of Breast Diseases

Eriko Tohno MD

Postdoctoral Fellow, University of Tsukuba, Tsukuba, Ibaraki, Japan

David O. Cosgrove MA MSc FRCR FRCP

Consultant in Nuclear Medicine and Ultrasound, Royal Postgraduate Medical School, Hammersmith Hospital, London, UK

John P. Sloane MB BS FRCPath

Consultant Histopathologist, Royal Marsden Hospital, Sutton, UK

with a contribution by

Efthiklis Vagios

Head of Department of Ultrasound and Mammography, 'Engephalos' Diagnostic Centre, Heraclion, Crete, Greece; Formerly Honorary Senior Registrar, Department of Nuclear Medicine and Ultrasound, Royal Marsden Hospital, London, UK

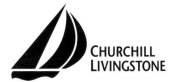

CHURCHILL
LIVINGSTONE

EDINBURGH LONDON MADRID MELBOURNE NEW YORK AND TOKYO 1994

CHURCHILL LIVINGSTONE
Medical Division of Pearson Professional Ltd

Distributed in the United States of America by Churchill Livingstone
Inc., 650 Avenue of the Americas, New York, N.Y. 10011, and by
associated companies, branches and representatives throughout the
world.

First published 1994
  Reprinted 1995
  Reprinted 1996

ISBN 0-443-04387-6

British Library of Cataloguing in Publication Data
A catalogue record for this book is available from the British Library.

Library of Congress Cataloging in Publication Data
Tohno, Eriko.
  Ultrasound diagnosis of breast diseases/Eriko Tohno, David O.
Cosgrove, John P. Sloane; with a contribution by Efthiklis Vagios.
      p. cm.
  Includes index.
  ISBN 0-443-04387-6
  1. Breast-Ultrasonic imaging. I. Cosgrove, David O.
II. Sloane, J.P. III. Title.
  [DNLM: 1. Breast Diseases-ultrasonography. WP 815 T645u 1993]
RG493.5.U47T64 1993
618.1'907543-dc20
DNLM/DLC
for Library of Congress   93-21522

Produced by Longman Singapore Publishers Pte Ltd.
Printed in Singapore

CONTENTS

Ultrasound has become a popular method for examining the breast. Increased general concern over breast diseases has reduced the number of women who attend breast clinics with large and clinically obvious carcinomas and increased those who attend with various symptoms, only some of whom actually have early carcinomas or other significant pathology. In addition, mammographic screening programmes, which are becoming implemented increasingly in many countries, reveal radiographically equivocal lesions that may be impalpable. On the other hand, avoidance of surgery for benign lesions is preferable on good clinical and economic grounds. Therefore accurate non-invasive diagnosis has become increasingly important.

Compared to the water-tank or water-bag systems, hand-held real-time transducers of high frequency have made ultrasound equipment cheaper, simplified the technique and shortened the examination time. Ultrasound is now available in many breast clinics and ultrasound departments; obviously a knowledge of breast ultrasound has become indispensable for those involved in breast diagnosis.

Ultrasound performed by skilled examiners with suitable equipment can detect small carcinomas less than 1 cm in diameter and diagnose a range of benign breast diseases accurately. On the other hand, because normal breast tissue is heterogeneous with variable ultrasonic patterns, ultrasound produces false positive results which could have the detrimental effect of increasing the benign biopsy rate. Significant abnormalities may be missed altogether. There are also important limitations for ultrasound, such as the difficulty in detection of micro-calcification and the overlap between some benign and malignant features, where the accuracy of other modalities, especially X-ray mammography, is superior.

Background knowledge of the general features of individual breast diseases, such as their incidence, age distribution, symptoms and palpatory features, is very important for correct ultrasound diagnosis. Sonographers examining the breast from a background of general ultrasound may not be familiar with these aspects so, in this textbook, the essential clinical features are described in each section. Those performing ultrasound as a part of integrated diagnosis who may not understand the physical and mechanical characteristics of ultrasound well may find the basis for interpreting images (described in Ch. 1) useful. Histological structure is the fundamental source of the images of ultrasound so the essential histopathological features of breast diseases are also described in each section, with an emphasis on the gross changes that are more important for ultrasonography than the fine detail which is of more interest to histopathologists.

The breast is a superficial organ so most breast carcinomas are palpable. A skilled clinician can distinguish between benign and malignant masses with high accuracy, but long personal experience of palpation is needed to develop this skill. Fortunately, in diagnostic imaging, experiences can be shared via the images produced. We hope this book will help and guide sonographers studying the breast to improve diagnosis and management of these often difficult and distressing diseases.

1993

E.T.
D.O.C.
J.P.S.

ACKNOWLEDGEMENTS

We gratefully acknowledge the indispensable help of Dr Jeff Bamber, who reviewed the chapter on the basic aspects of ultrasound, and of Dr Jane Davey and Mr Alan McKinna, both of whom advised extensively on clinical aspects.

Dr Tohno was partly funded by a grant from the CRC/ICR during her stay at the Royal Marsden Hospital; it was the practical support and patient encouragement of Professor Kit Hill that allowed this book to be written.

David Cosgrove extends particular thanks to Sam and Lu Maslak for their encouragement and support in addressing and extending the potential for ultrasound diagnosis in breast diseases.

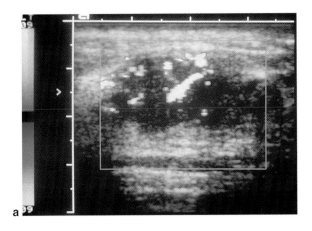 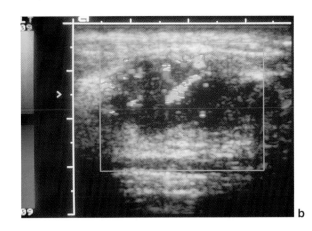

a   b

Plate C.1
Colour Doppler
The vessels in and around a breast carcinoma are displayed as colour Doppler signals. The direction of blood flow is encoded according to the colour bar alongside the image, with colours above the black baseline band (red in this example (**a**)) indicating flow towards the transducer and colours below the base-line (blue in this example) indicating flow away from the transducer. The velocity is encoded as saturation of the colours. Decreased saturation (lighter colour) indicates higher Doppler shift due to high flow velocity. The particular colours used may be changed or inverted, the choice being largely a matter of user preference. Another popular colour combination (**b**) shows shades of different hues (red-to-yellow and blue-to-green).

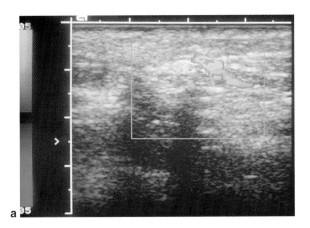 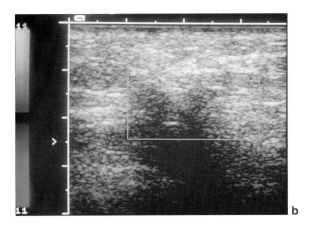

a   b

Plate C.2
Aliasing on colour Doppler
On colour Doppler, the aliasing artefact shows as a mosaic of different colours without a black band separating each block of colour (**a**). It can be removed by raising the velocity scale but only at the expense of loss of sensitivity, so that fewer colour signals are shown (**b**). In practice, aliasing is not often encountered because the flow velocity with the small normal breast or tumour vessels is rarely high enough to cause the problem.

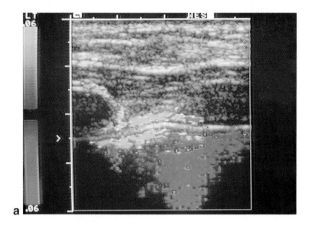 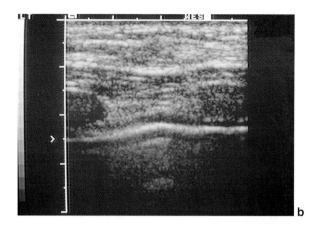

Plate C.3
Mirror image artefact
Two vessels running parallel to each other are seen in the parasternal area (**a**). The deeper is a mirror image artefact, caused by strong reflection at the lung surface; the same effect is also apparent on the B-mode image (**b**). (The intense blue band deeper in the scan is a motion artefact produced by pleural motion during breathing.)

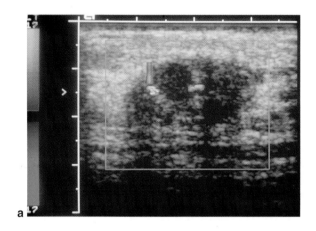 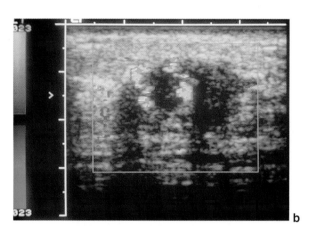

Plate C.4
Colour capture
Only a small proportion of the vessels that are actually present in the region of tissue being examined can be visualised on a frozen image because it is an instantaneous still frame of a thin slice (**a**). Using 'colour capture' the colour signals acquired over a preset time (4 s is usually chosen) are accumulated to form the final display so that more of the vascular activity is represented. In addition, the transducer can be scanned slowly across the lesion during the accumulation period to project the three-dimensional arrangements of the vessels onto one plane, so that tortuous vessels are seen as continuous lines (**b**).

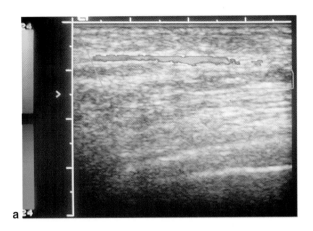

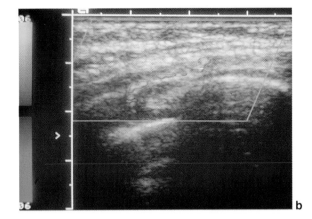

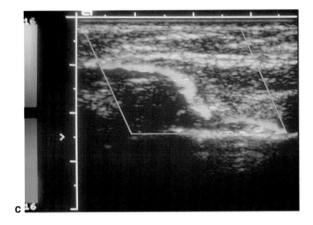

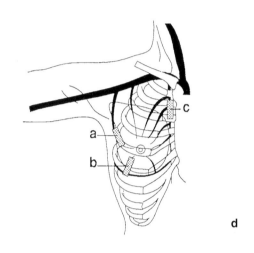

Plate C.5
Arteries of the breast
a. A lateral mammary branch from the lateral thoracic artery.
b. A perforating branch from the intercostal artery.
c. A perforating branch from the internal mammary artery.
d. Line diagram showing position of scans **a–c**.

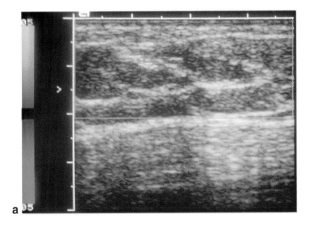

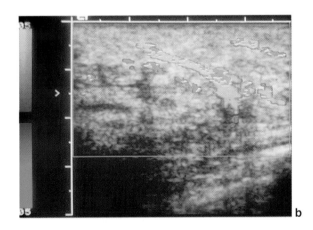

Plate C.6
Normal vessels within the breast
a. The arteries of the normal breast often run along the Cooper's ligaments.
b. Increased vascularity in a pregnant breast.

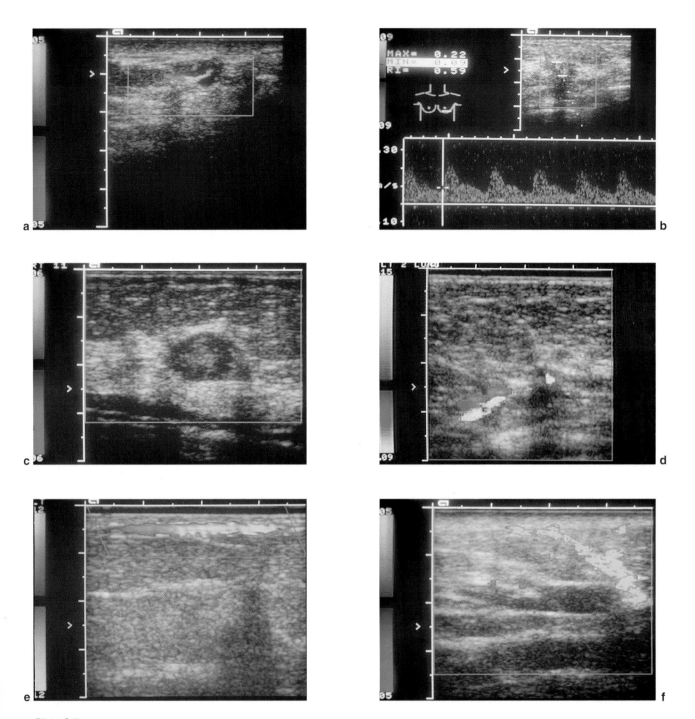

Plate C.7
Breast carcinomas

a. Increased vascularity is seen in most breast carcinomas, even those that are small (this was an 8 mm lesion). Feeding vessels form at the edge of the tumour or in the adjacent breast tissue and grow into the mass.

b. Spectral analysis is facilitated by colour Doppler because the sensitive gate can be located precisely on one of the vessels. The Doppler spectrum typically shows continuous diastolic flow (RI=0.59, a low resistance pattern) though this is not always the case with breast carcinomas.

c. Vessels within a mass are suspicious even when the lesion has a benign appearance on the scan. This lesion which seemed innocent on real-time imaging but was vascular, proved to be a carcinoma on histology.

d. Occasionally, increased vascularity indicates the presence of a small carcinoma that would otherwise be difficult to detect.

e. A dilated subcutaneous vein draining an advanced breast carcinoma. Subcutaneous veins are seen just under the skin and run parallel to it. (Same case as Fig. 4.19.)

f. Inflammatory carcinoma. Many vessels of high velocity are seen in the subcutaneous fat layer.

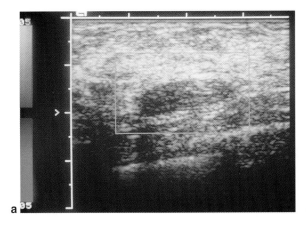
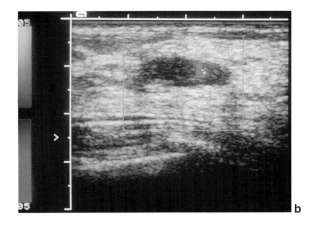

a   b

Plate C.8
Fibroadenomas
a. Usually no vessels are seen in association with fibroadenomas.
b. Doppler signals were obtained from this lesion. Some 20% of fibroadenomas are vascular, especially those of large size and those developing in young women.

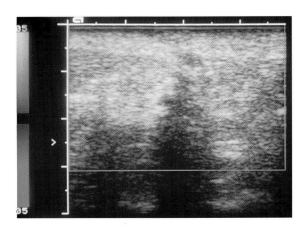
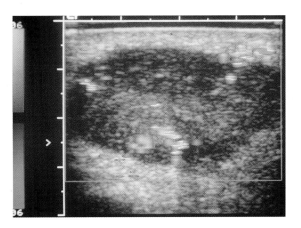

Plate C.9
Benign breast change
No colour Doppler signals are seen in this area of architectural change. Benign breast change is usually avascular though some cases, where there is an inflammatory component, do contain blood vessels.

Plate C.10
Phylloides tumour
Several vessels are seen within this mass. Although this appearance is not specific for malignancy, it suggests an actively growing tumour. (Same case as Fig. 5.14.)

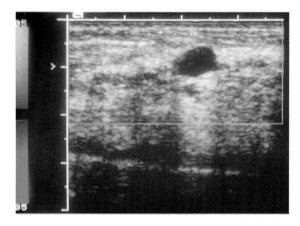

Plate C.11
Cyst
Cysts are always avascular. Any deviation from this rule is suspicious.

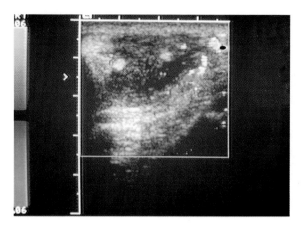

Plate C.12
Abscess
A marked increase in vascularity is observed in the wall and surrounding tissue of a breast abscess. (Same case as Fig. 7.2.b.)

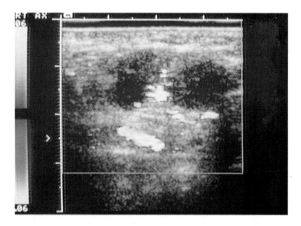

Plate C.13
Colour Doppler positive metastatic axillary lymph nodes
Engorged vessels with high velocity flow are seen around these metastatic lymph nodes. (Same lesion as Fig.10.2.a.)

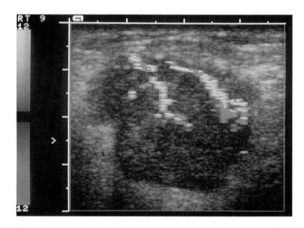

Plate C.14
Metastatic melanoma in breast
Very prominent, flame-like vascularity is seen in this lesion. This pattern is characteristic of a melanoma, whether primary or secondary. (Same case as Fig.10.5.)

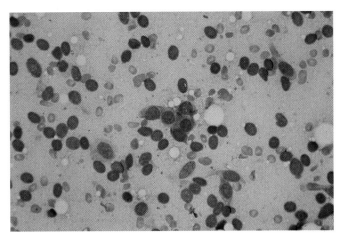

Plate P.2.1
Cytological smear of a fine needle aspirate of a fibroadenoma
The cell nuclei are fairly uniform in size and staining intensity; there are many ovoid 'bare' nuclei devoid of cytoplasm which are derived from myoepithelial cells. The presence of such nuclei in a breast aspirate is strongly in favour of a benign diagnosis. The anucleate green-staining cells in the background are red blood cells. (Giemsa; ×286.)

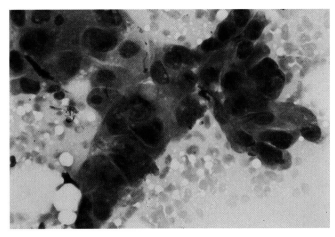

Plate P.2.2
Cytological smear of a fine needle aspirate of an infiltrating ductal carcinoma
There is a clump of cells with very large nuclei which vary considerably in shape, size and staining intensity; many contain prominent nucleoli. No myoepithelial cells are present. (Giemsa; ×286.)

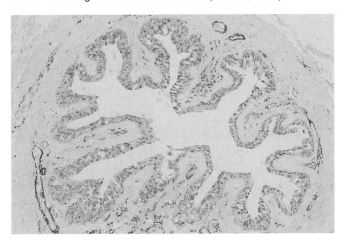

Plate P.3.1.
Histology of normal breast
Section of a major subareolar duct (lactiferous sinus) which has been stained by the immunoalkaline phosphatase technique to highlight the contractile protein actin. Note the outer myoepithelial cells with actin positive (red) cytoplasm and the inner epithelial cells which do not take up the red stain. The small blood vessels around the duct are also positive. Lactiferous sinuses have an important role in storing milk during lactation; the infolding of the walls allows for the marked expansion necessary to perform this function. (×65.)

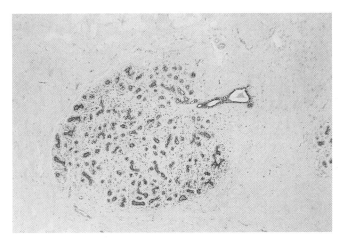

Plate P.3.2.
Normal terminal duct lobular unit
The acini are surrounded by stroma which is more cellular and loosely textured than that outside the lobule. The extralobular terminal duct is seen on the upper right of the picture. (×26.)

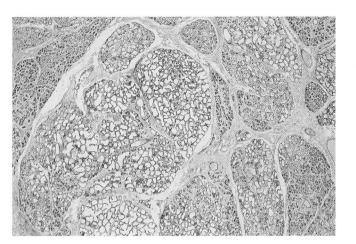

Plate P.3.3.
Lactating breast
The terminal duct lobular units are massively enlarged and their acini dilated with secretion. The pink staining collagenous interlobular stroma is extensively obliterated. (×13.)

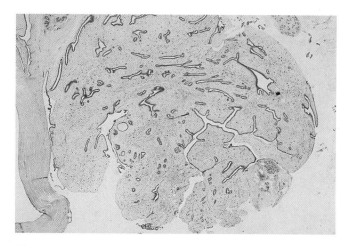

Plate P.5.1
Histological patterns in fibroadenomas
This fibroadenoma exhibits a pericanalicular growth pattern at the top left of the picture and an intracanalicular pattern at the bottom right. The capsule is seen on the left but has become separated from the rest of the lesion (a preparation artefact). (×13.)

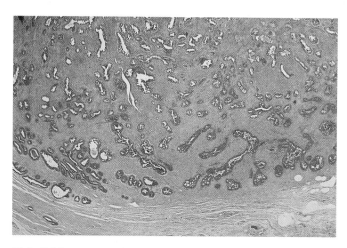

Plate P.5.2
Juvenile fibroadenoma
The lesion has a circumscribed edge seen at the bottom of the picture. The epithelial component is very cellular and takes the form of numerous duct-like structures with intraluminal proliferation. The intervening stroma is also very cellular but this feature is not readily seen at this magnification. (×26.)

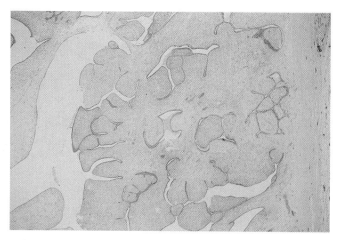

Plate P.5.3
Phylloides tumour
Phylloides tumour with an intracanalicular growth pattern demonstrating the characteristic leaf-like processes projecting into a cystic space on the left of the picture. (×26.)

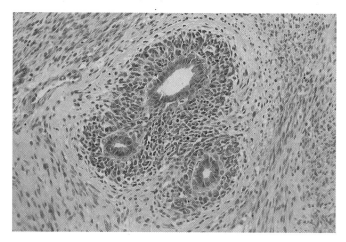

Plate P.5.4
Phylloides tumour (magnified view)
A high power view of a high grade phylloides tumour showing three glandular structures surrounded by densely cellular stroma composed of cytologically malignant cells which are rounder next to the epithelium and more spindle-shaped elsewhere. The growth pattern here is pericanalicular. (×65.)

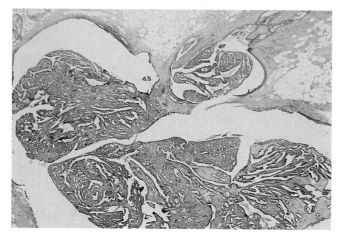

Plate P.5.5
Intracystic papilloma
The tumour has well-developed papillae with fibrovascular cores and lies within a cystically dilated duct. (×13.)

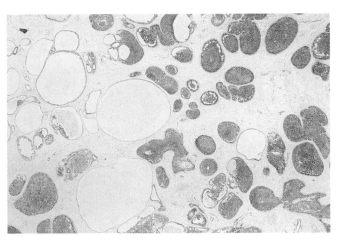

Plate P.5.6
Juvenile papillomatosis
There are numerous acini and ducts with cystic dilatation (mostly on the left) and solid intraluminal proliferation (mostly on the right). Sclerosing adenosis is not seen in this example. (×13.)

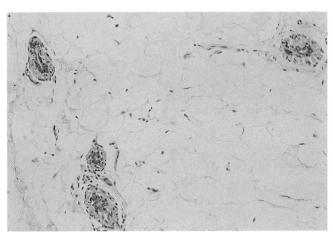

Plate P.5.7
Adenolipoma
Several small normal-looking glandular structures are separated by normal adipocytes which have voluminous clear cytoplasm and faintly defined cell borders. (×65.)

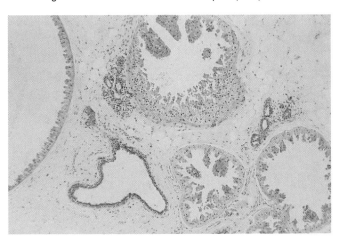

Plate P.6.1
Histology of simple cysts
There are several cysts lined by cells which have the characteristic apocrine metaplasia. The large cyst on the left is generally lined by a single layer of cells but the others show papillary tufting. Most of the apparent hyperplasia in the lower half of the top cyst, however, is due to tangential cutting. Note for comparison the normal interlobular duct in the lower half of the picture and remnants of two terminal duct lobular units in the centre. (×26.)

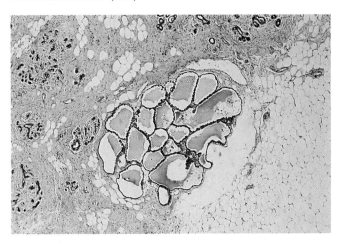

Plate P.6.2
Lactational focus
In the centre of the picture is a grossly enlarged terminal duct lobular unit exhibiting secretory changes indistinguishable from that seen in pregnancy and lactation. Note the normal units in the left and upper parts of the picture for comparison. (×13.)

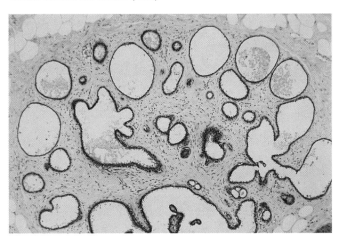

Plate P.6.3
Blunt duct adenosis
This terminal duct lobular unit has formed cysts that are much smaller than those seen in Plate P.6.1, embedded in specialised cellular stroma. (×10.)

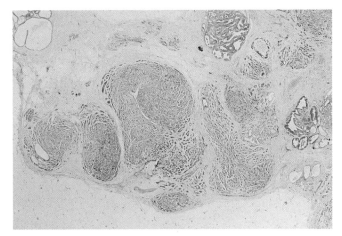

Plate P.6.4
Sclerosing adenosis
There is gross enlargement of the terminal duct lobular units in the centre of the picture due to a marked increase in the number of acini which have spiky, infiltrative outlines. A few small cysts are also present in this illustration. (×13.)

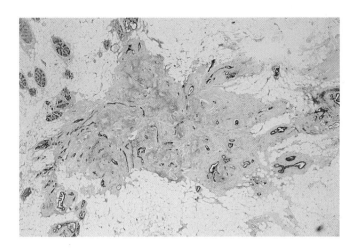

Plate P.6.5
Radial scar
There is a stellate zone of fibrosis and elastosis, the latter appearing as more deeply stained irregular pink material distributed thoughout the fibrous tissue. Irregular infiltrative-looking glandular structures are scattered througout the fibroelastotic tissue. The proportion of the stroma is unusually prominent — perhaps related to the age of the lesion. (×26.)

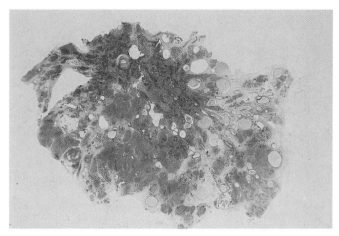

Plate P.6.6
Complex sclerosing lesion
There is a small fibroelastotic zone at the top left of the picture (only part of the lesion is included in this section) from which radiate out numerous terminal duct lobular units exhibiting sclerosing adenosis and cyst formation. Other examples of this condition show a higher ratio of stroma to epithelium. This lesion and the radial scar illustrated in Plate P.6.5 represent extremes in terms of the relative proportions of stroma and epithelium. (×26.)

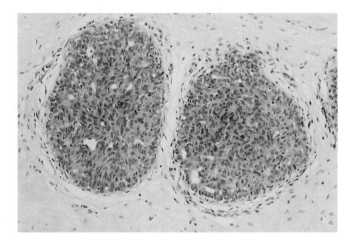

Plate P.6.7
Hyperplasia of usual type
Two acini are grossly distended and occluded by intraluminal proliferation of epithelial cells which lack cytological evidence of malignancy and are accompanied by myoepithelial cells and leucocytes. Nuclear spacing is very uneven and the secondary lumina are indistinct. (×65.)

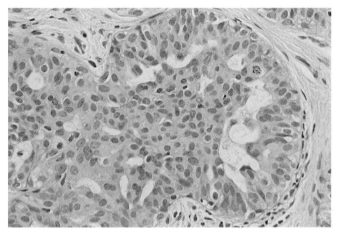

Plate P.6.8
Atypical ductal hyperplasia
The picture shows an interlobular duct at high magnification. In this example, there is a mixture of epithelial cells, myoepithelial cells (with smaller, more darkly staining ovoid nuclei) and leucocytes (small, round, darkly staining nuclei) as seen in hyperplasia of usual type. The epithelial cells, however, show some cytological atypia with nuclei that vary in size, shape and staining intensity. A mitosis is seen at the top right of the picture. (×65.)

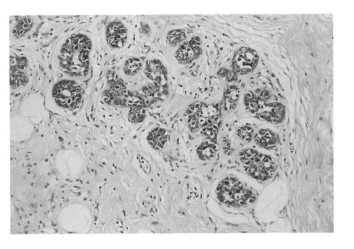

Plate P.6.9
Atypical lobular hyperplasia
A terminal duct lobular unit exhibits intraluminal proliferation of small uniform, uncohesive cells identical in appearance to those seen in lobular carcinoma in situ. The appearances fall short of malignancy because the distension of acini is minor, the lumina are focally preserved and there is a mixture of cell types. (×65.)

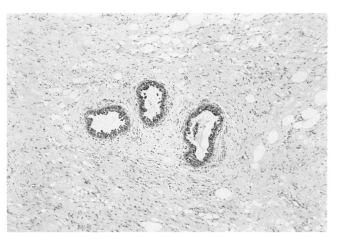

Plate P.6.10
Gynaecomastia, active phase
Three ducts show significant intraluminal papillary proliferation but without complete occlusion. The surrounding stroma is hypercellular due to proliferation of fibroblasts which have replaced many of the fat cells. Terminal duct lobular units are not normally present in the male breast and only very rarely appear in gynaecomastia. (×65.)

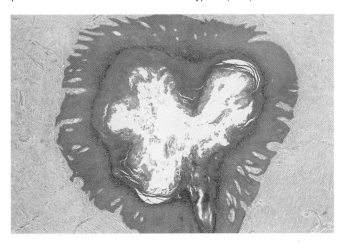

Plate P.7.1
Recurring subareolar abscess
The section shows a major subareolar duct with squamous metaplasia and occlusion of the lumen by keratin and cornified epithelial cells. No significant inflammation was present around the duct itself at the time of excision. (×26.)

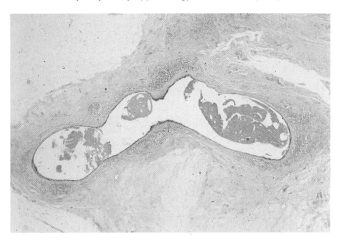

Plate P.7.2
Major duct ectasia
A large dilated subareolar duct is distended with homogeneous, deeply eosinophilic (pink) secretion and surrounded by a dense infiltrate of chronic inflammatory cells which appear as a collection of dark blue dots in this low power illustration. (×26.)

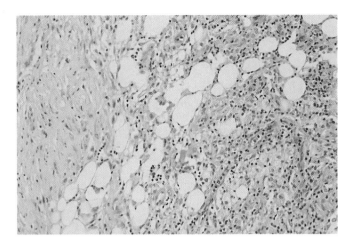

Plate P.8.1
Fat necrosis
A few residual adipocytes can be seen in the centre and on the right of the picture. They are mixed with many lymphocytes and histiocytes with vacuolated cytoplasm. A few multinucleate giant cells are present. A zone of fibrosis can be seen on the left. (×65.)

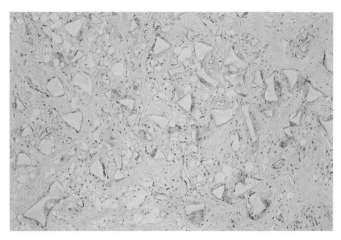

Plate P.8.2
Reaction to silicone prosthesis
Many irregular fragments of the prosthetic material are directly surrounded by foreign body giant cells. The intervening breast tissue shows fibrosis and collections of silicone-containing macrophages. (×26.)

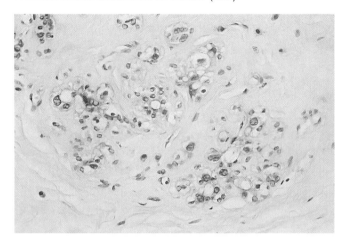

Plate P.8.3
Irradiation change
A terminal duct lobular unit showing loss of acini and fibrous replacement. Some of the epithelial cells have been lost and some of the remainder contain large, densely staining nuclei which might be mistaken for malignancy if the history of irradiation is not known. (×143.)

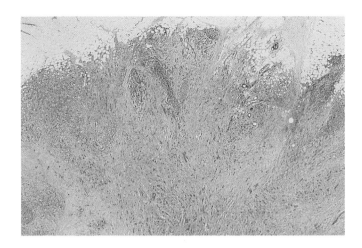

Plate P.9.1
Invasive ductal carcinoma
This low power view shows the irregular edge of the tumour where it infiltrates the fibroadipose tissue in the upper half of the picture. Much of the tumour consists of pink-staining fibrous tissue in which are embedded small islands of malignant epithelial cells of variable size and shape. Aggregates of chronic inflammatory cells are also seen. (×13.)

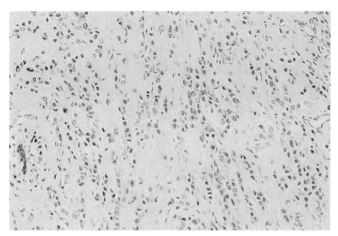

Plate P.9.2
Invasive lobular carcinoma
This high power view shows two characteristic histological features of the classical form of this type of breast carcinoma: (1) the small round tumour cells with high nucleus/cytoplasm ratio and (2) their pattern of infiltration either as single cells or in lines known as 'Indian files'. (×65.)

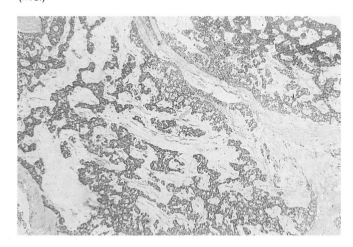

Plate P.9.3
Colloid carcinoma
Irregular interconnecting masses of rather small regular tumour cells are surrounded by lakes of mucin. (×26.)

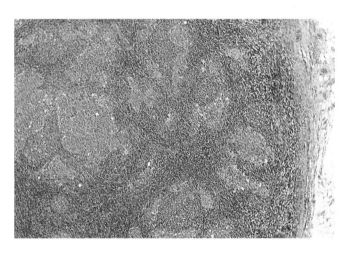

Plate P.9.4
Medullary carcinoma
This low power view shows the degree of circumscription with the border of the tumour on the right. The irregular pinker zones are the malignant epithelial cells and the darker, bluer areas are the infiltrating chronic inflammatory cells. (×13.)

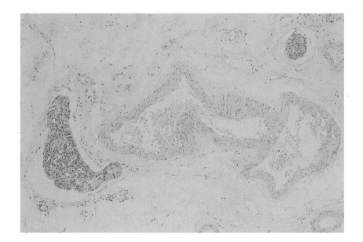

Plate P.9.5
Inflammatory carcinoma
Tumour emboli within lymphatic vessels are seen at the bottom left and top right of the picture and accompanying large blood vessel is present in the centre. (×65.)

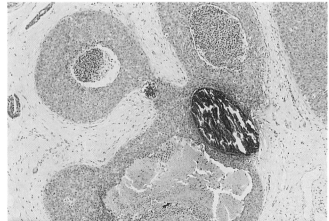

Plate P.9.6
Ductal carcinoma in situ, comedo type
A duct is grossly distended with large malignant cells which have undergone central necrosis in three places. A large focus of calcification (staining purple with haematoxylin) is seen in the central part of the picture. (×26.)

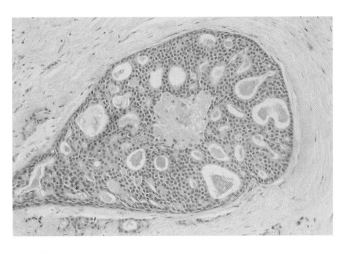

Plate P.9.7
Ductal carcinoma in situ, cribriform type
Note the sieve-like growth pattern in which the well-delineated lumina are separated by a monomorphic population of tumour cells. Compared with the comedo variant, the tumour cells have smaller, rounder, more densely staining nuclei with a higher nucleus/cytoplasm ratio. (×65.)

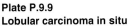

Plate P.9.8
Ductal carcinoma in situ, micropapillary type
The cells are similar to those seen in the cribriform variant but are arranged in papillae, some of which have fibrovascular cores (right). On the left there is fusion of papillae to produce the so-called 'Roman bridges'. (×143.)

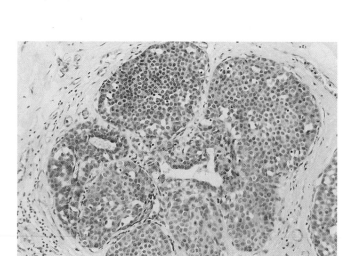

Plate P.9.9
Lobular carcinoma in situ
This high power view shows moderate distension of the acini in one terminal duct lobular unit by a solid proliferation of small uniform, rounded cells with high nucleus/cytoplasm ratio. The lack of cellular cohesion is characteristic. The cells may be mistaken for those of the cribriform/papillary variant of ductal carcinoma in situ but are distinguished by their growth pattern and intracytoplasmic mucin globules which can be demonstrated with histochemical stains. (×143.)

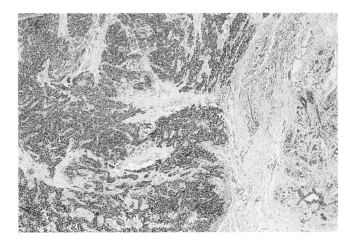

Plate P.10.1
Metastatic lung cancer
Metastatic deposit in the breast arising from a small cell anaplastic ('oat cell') carcinoma of the bronchus. The tumour is seen on the left of the picture and a few residual terminal duct lobular units on the right. (×26.)

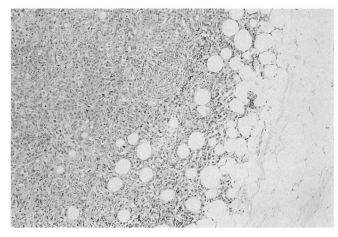

Plate P.10.2
Primary diffuse, large cell, malignant lymphoma of the breast
The relative sparing of fat spaces around the infiltrative edge of the tumour is a characteristic feature of lymphomas. (×26.)

Chapter 1

Basic aspects of ultrasound

Ultrasound is now well established as an important technique for the investigation of breast problems. It is a curious fact that, although breast diagnosis was one of the earliest clinical applications of ultrasound, its widespread use has been considerably delayed. This is attributable partly to the success of X-ray mammography, but also to the difficulties of using ultrasound in the breast because of its complex anatomy with an abundance of fat which disturbs the pattern of the ultrasound beam thus degrading the quality of the scans. These problems have largely been resolved as an improved understanding of the anatomy and of the relevant ultrasound physics has led to the development of more appropriate ultrasound scanners.

In this chapter the basic principles of diagnostic ultrasound are described with an emphasis on the applications in the breast, together with a description of the main types of equipment that have been developed for this purpose. This survey is of interest not only for historical reasons but also because the sequence of developments underlines the numerous technical problems of ultrasound mammography which each new type of scanner was designed to resolve. It is the creative use of the experience derived from these attempts and the enrichment of the morphological examination with functional information provided by Doppler that has led to the current high reliability of ultrasound mammography using multipurpose real-time, high resolution scanners. All of the clinical images presented in this book have been obtained using such state-of-the-art equipment. Experimental techniques, such as the C-scan and computed ultrasound tomography, have been omitted since they have not found routine application.

EQUIPMENT

The first investigations of the role of ultrasound for the breast were by Wild and Reid in the early 1950s, using a direct contact A-mode system operating at 15 MHz. The tip of the transducer was covered with a small water-bag to separate the transducer from the skin so as to avoid imaging in the very near field where the beam was subject to distortions. Further developments of this technique (reported in 1952) indicated that it was possible to distinguish between benign and malignant breast lesions[1]. Howry et al[2] were the first to use a B-mode scanner, publishing the first ultrasound images of a schirrous carcinoma in a mastectomy specimen using a water-bath scanner in 1954.

The early 15 MHz hand-held B-scanner of Wild, in fact, provided near real-time images by repeating the frames at a high rate. After many more-or-less successful water-bath scanners, both compound and single-pass, developed by Japanese, Australian and other American investigators, history has turned full circle with the general reversion to a direct contact approach some using a stand-off device, but now giving real-time imaging. Modern hand-held real-time transducers, particularly mechanical sector designs that are equipped with a small water-bag, are very similar to Wild's scanner. The main differences are the use of a lower frequency (15 MHz could not penetrate more than about 2 cm into the breast), better spatial resolution (Wild's transducer was not focused), a faster frame rate for better real-time, the use of a scan converter and a wide dynamic range for gray-scale display.

Compound scans

A compound scan is formed by summing multiple single-pass scans onto the same image, overlapping the information obtained from different lines of sight (Fig. 1.1.a). It has the advantage of providing a complete display of boundaries, and ductal structures are well displayed in either cross- or longitudinal sections[3], but these scanners are complex and cannot provide real-time imaging. In addition, the image quality is degraded by refraction due to the low velocity of ultrasound in fat that causes misregistration of structures imaged from the different directions. Because of these problems, this approach has been abandoned, after a substantial period of popularity, during which several commercial systems dedicated to breast scanning were marketed.

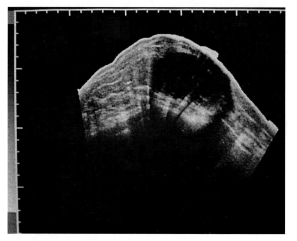
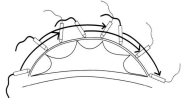

Fig. 1.1
Methods for breast imaging
a. Direct contact compound method. The image is formed by summing multiple scans. The angle can be changed to optimise the imaging of interfaces at different angles. The whole breast is visualised on a single image and the margins of lesions are well-displayed (a breast abscess in this case).

b. Water-bath method with the patient supine. The patient lies supine with the water-bath placed on the breast. The single transducer is moved mechanically to form an image in either a linear or arc configuration. The breast is flattened by the water-bag so that the whole breast is within the focal zone and the lesion (breast carcinoma, arrow) is clearly demonstrated.

c. Water-bath scan with the patient prone (Octoson). The patient lies prone with the breast immersed in a water-tank. Sector movements of each transducer form single-pass images which are combined into a compound scan. The whole margin of a cyst (arrow) at the periphery of the breast is well-displayed. Although the patient is scanned supine, the images are usually presented upside-down to correspond with scans from other systems. (Image kindly supplied by Dr. W.R . Hateley of the Royal London Hospital.)

d. Real-time mechanical sector scan. A simple transducer in a small water-bag moves rapidly in an arc to form real-time images with a triangular or trapezoidal shape. The position of the scan can be adjusted so that the region of interest (breast carcinoma, the same case as **b**) is centred in the image.

e. Real-time electronic linear scan. An array of transducer elements is switched to create real-time images with a rectangular shape. Flexibility of

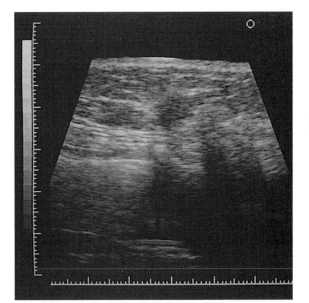
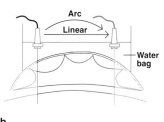

b

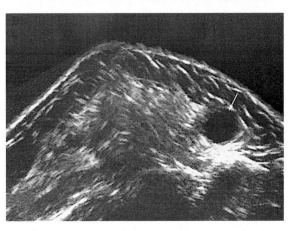
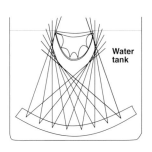

c

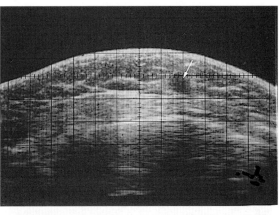
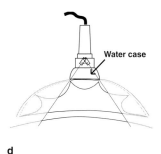

d

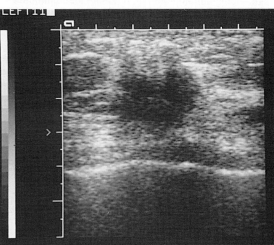
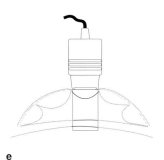

e

Automatic water-bath scanners

Several dedicated automatic breast scanners have been developed over the past few decades. The term 'automatic' implies ease of use but, in reality, these systems demanded considerable skill and experience on the part of the operator both for patient positioning and for machine settings[4]. An attraction of this approach was that serial images of the entire breast could be produced in multiple planes so that its internal architecture was well displayed. It was claimed that the scanning technique and image interpretation were easier and more reproducible than with hand-held systems[5]. Another argument in favour of dedicated breast scanners is the reduced operator dependence; it is true that this remains a problem with hand-held systems, which were deemed valuable only for the study of focal regions of interest and not suitable for screening programmes. Several different approaches were available for automatic systems operating with the patient prone, supine or in the sitting position.

In 1950 the Japanese group of Kikuchi et al[6] described one of the first scanners of this type, operating with the patient supine. An unfocused 5 MHz transducer was used with a water-bag. By the 1960s the limitations of unfocused transducers were recognised and improved units using focused transducers were developed[7].

Jellins and Kossoff in Australia in 1966 developed a specialised scanner consisting of a large water-tank on which the patient lay with both breasts immersed. A large aperture (f.25) 2 MHz transducer gave a range resolution of 1 mm (2 mm laterally). In the first version the breasts were compressed by a plastic sheet, a later modification allowing imaging either with or without compression[8,9]. Gray-scale display was also introduced at this time. In 1960 Kelly-Fry[10] developed a similar system that was controlled by a computer.

In 1969 Deland[11] described a scanner using an unfocused 2.25 MHz 12 mm transmitting transducer whose aperture is further reduced to 6 mm by a cork collimator. Four receiving transducers were used to improve lateral resolution. The patient was scanned with the breasts uncompressed in a water-bath.

A closed water-bath system was developed in 1976 by Wagai[12] (Fig. 1.1.b). The patient lay supine with the transducer located over one quadrant. Scanning was automated with a mechanical driver to obtain a series of images at spaced distances. The scan head had to be repositioned to examine other quadrants of the breast. The echo patterns of both carcinomas and benign breast lesions were described.

In 1976 Kossoff et al[13] described a new multipurpose water-bath scanner using eight single-focus transducers appropriately named the Octoson (Fig. 1.1.c). The transducers were mounted on a movable frame in a large water-tank with mechanical linkages to provide both single-pass sector and compound scanning. After attempts using various combinations, transducers of 7 cm in diameter operating at 3 MHz were adopted. The system produced images with an excellent gray-scale and good resolution while the repeatability of scan planes was a major advantage. The Octoson did much to raise awareness to the potential of ultrasound for breast examination before the advent of modern sophisticated real-time systems.

A hybrid scanner was developed by Foster[14] in 1983 using a 5 cm five element annular array operating at 4 MHz for transmission. The echoes were received by a very wide aperture (37.5 cm) conical transducer which gave extremely good resolution. The size of the receiver dictated a water-bath approach.

A scanner for use in the sitting position was developed by Baum in the 1970s. A particular feature of this system was that the breast was not compressed on the supposition that external compression would modify the internal texture of the gland, with an adverse effect on lesion detectability. The system used a 2.25 MHz transducer with a television-based method for quantitation of the gray-scale on the image and displaying it with colour coding. Subsequent improvements[15] allowed scanning in multiple directions and also provided arc scanning. In a further development of the arc scanning modality, the transducer was placed to allow the focal zone of the beam to follow the shape of the uncompressed breast in a parabola.

Real-time scanners

Real-time transducers were introduced for cardiac and abdominal applications much earlier than for the breast, presumably because the display of tissue movement is much more important in these areas. Early transducers could only be used to guide biopsies because they produced poor images with limited spatial resolution since they operated at a low frequency and were unfocused. The loss of textural detail was obvious by comparison with the images obtained from dedicated water-bath systems. However, during the early 1980s, high resolution real-time transducers were developed for superficial organs (e.g. the eye, thyroid and testis). The image quality was at least comparable to that obtained from dedicated water-bath systems and they had the practical advantage of forming part of general purpose ultrasound scanners and thus being cheaper. The benefits of the real-time direct contact approach are overwhelming, despite some disadvantages[16–18] (Table 1.1) and the wide availability of these systems accounts in part for the increasing application of ultrasound for breast diagnosis.

Table 1.1 Static vs. real-time scanners		
	Static	**Real-time**
Field of view	Wide	Small
Comparison with the opposite side or previous examination	Good	Difficult
Examination time	Long	Short
Price	High	Low–medium
Patient positioning	Elaborate	Simple
Dynamic tests	Unsuitable	Easy
Interventional techniques	Difficult	Simple

Several types of real-time system are suitable for breast ultrasound. Mechanical scanners produce high quality images by moving a single ultrasound transducer rapidly over the region of interest (Fig. 1.1.d). Electronic scanners use an array of transducer elements which are switched serially to form and move the ultrasound beam (Fig. 1.1.e). They have the additional advantages of a sharp focus throughout the depth of the image and of providing a platform to which Doppler is easily added, whereas with mechanical systems this is difficult. A shallow stand-off is often used to locate the glandular tissue of the breast at the focal zone, particularly for mechanical systems, where it is convenient to have the stand-off incorporated into the transducer itself, especially for interventional procedures. In modern electronic systems the resolution is maintained to within a millimetre or so of the transducer surface and so they are generally used without a stand-off, except when the skin itself or very superficial lesions must be imaged.

BASIC ASPECTS OF ULTRASOUND

Sound whose frequency is higher than the upper limit of audibility (nominally taken as 20 kHz, a hertz being one cycle per second) is defined as 'ultrasound'. Because the spatial resolution in an ultrasound image is proportional to the frequency used, as high a frequency as possible is preferred for imaging; however, attenuation of ultrasound by the tissues it traverses increases in proportion to frequency and so a compromise has to be reached. In practice, for breast examinations frequencies in the 5–10 MHz range are suitable, with 7.5 MHz being most often chosen.

Ultrasound is generated by a transducer which converts electrical energy into ultrasound energy. The conversion is effected by piezoelectric materials which have the property that a change of voltage across the surfaces causes the material to change thickness. Since the effect is symmetrical (i.e. a change in thickness of the transducer material produces a voltage across its surfaces) the same transducer can be used as an ultrasound receiver. The most commonly used piezoelectric material is lead zirconate titanate; more recently, polyvinylidene fluoride, a synthetic plastic, has been introduced.

Both audible sound and ultrasound are mechanical waves that are conducted through materials whose particles are alternately compressed and rarefied; since the particles move in the same direction as the overall propagation of the wave, this is termed a 'longitudinal wave' in contradistinction to a ripple on the surface of a pool which is a 'transverse wave' because the water molecules move up and down while the wave travels horizontally. The wavelength, which determines the best range resolution that can be obtained, is inversely proportional to the ultrasound frequency; at 7.5 MHz the wavelength is approximately 0.2 mm. The velocity of ultrasound is almost constant at 1540 m/s in soft tissue.

Echo production and conduction

The basis of diagnostic ultrasound scanning, the 'pulse-echo' method, is the reflection of a portion of the transmitted ultrasound back towards its source when it strikes a surface. To form an image both the direction and the depth of each surface must be determined: the direction of the ultrasound beam is known from the scanning action, while the depth can be calculated from the delay between transmission of the sound pulse and receipt of the echo, on the assumption that the velocity is constant. The same principle is used in RADAR and SONAR.

The ultrasound pulse is reflected whenever the beam crosses an interface between two adjacent tissues with different 'acoustic impedance' values. The impedance (Z) is determined by the density (ρ) and the velocity (c) of propagation of ultrasound through the tissue, the impedance being equal to density multiplied by velocity ($Z = \rho c$).

Two main types of echo are encountered clinically, depending on the structure of the reflecting surface. Where this is smooth relative to the ultrasound wavelength, Snell's law for refraction and reflection is obeyed and echoes are returned at an angle equal to the angle of incidence; this is known as 'specular' or mirror-like reflection by analogy with an optical mirror. In the breast, strong reflections of this type occur from the interfaces between subcutaneous fat and glandular parenchyma and from the margins of a mass. On the other hand, when the beam encounters an interface that is irregular, with a roughness the same order of size as the ultrasound wavelength itself, a different echo-producing mechanism occurs whereby the ultrasound is reflected or scattered equally in all directions. These scattered echoes are weak and typically arise from the soft tissue parenchyma itself (breast lobules, arterioles, etc.) and from the fine structure of solid lesions.

Attenuation

The ultrasound beam undergoes continuous modification during its passage through body tissues; the most important of these is attenuation which leads a progressive decrease in its intensity. Attenuation results from a combination of absorption, reflection and scattering, the first usually being dominant. Absorption occurs when the orderly particle movement characteristic of ultrasound is converted to random vibration which represents heat; it is approximately proportional to the number of large molecules present. Attenuation increases with increasing frequency, averaging 1 dB/cm MHz^{-1} for soft tissues. The amplitude of a 7.5 MHz ultrasound beam is attenuated by over 50% for every centimetre of depth penetrated. In order to maintain an approximate correspondence between image brightness and echo intensity, this loss is corrected in the ultrasound scanner by increasing the amplification with depth; the time gain compensating (TGC) amplifier performs this important function (Fig. 1.2). If a lesion absorbs more than the surrounding soft tissue for which the TGC has been adjusted, the tissue deep to the lesion appears darker. This is known as 'shad-

Fig. 1.2
Attenuation
The ultrasound beam is attenuated as it travels through tissue. To compensate for this the received signals are progressively amplified in proportion to their depth (i.e. the delay in their return) to display homogeneous tissue with equal intensity with depth (TGC, time gain compensation) (**a**).
If a lesion causes more attenuation than the adjacent tissues, the TGC correction is insufficient to compensate for the attenuation and so the echoes deep to the lesion are displayed as less intense than the adjacent tissues at the same depth, producing an acoustic shadow (**b**).
If ultrasound is attenuated less in a lesion than in the normal structures, the TGC overcompensates so that the signals behind the lesion are displayed as more intense than the surrounding structures, producing acoustic enhancement (**c**).

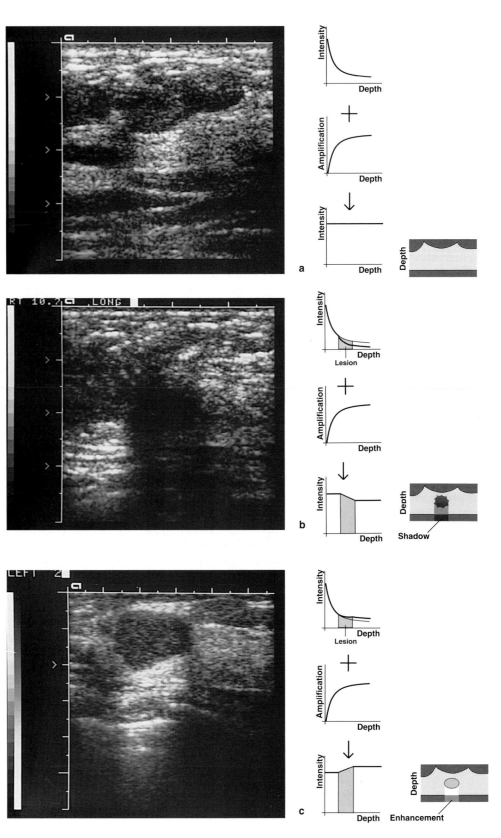

owing' and is typically found behind breast carcinomas. On the other hand, echoes behind a lesion which attenuates the ultrasound less are overcompensated and so appear more intense than the surrounding tissue, an effect known as acoustic 'enhancement' which is typical of cysts.

The ultrasound beam

A simple disc transducer produces an ultrasound beam whose diameter varies with distance from the transducer (Fig. 1.3). The diameter of the beam determines lateral resolution and so, for diagnostic use, it is narrowed by focusing. While focusing improves the resolution within the focal zone, it causes it to deteriorate superficially and deep to this region. Various methods such as concave shaping of the transducer surface, the addition of acoustic lenses or the use of complex multielement transducers (phased arrays) are employed, often in combination (Fig. 1.4). In practice the lateral resolution usually remains worse than axial resolution which is determined by the pulse length.

Fig. 1.3
The ultrasound beam
The shape of the ultrasound beam from a single-element disc transducer changes with depth, being wider away from the focal zone. The beam width determines the lateral resolution of the scan.

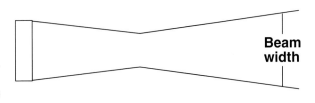

Fig. 1.4
Focusing
To improve lateral resolution, the ultrasound beam is focused either by curving the face of the transducer (**a**), using an acoustic lens (**b**) or by triggering the elements of an array with small time differences (electronic focusing, **c**). A penalty of focusing is that the beam becomes wider deep to the focal zone.

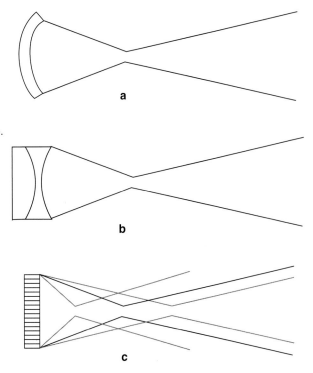

Doppler

Doppler has emerged as a promising addition to imaging in the detection and differential diagnosis of breast problems because the periphery of malignant lesions is vascularised while most benign processes are hypovascular, a notable exception being inflammatory lesions. Research into tumour vasculature began early in this century with the technique of injecting a mixture of bismuth and oil into the arteries supplying human cancers; radiographs of these specimens revealed abundant vasculature[19,20]. Malignant tumours larger than a few millimetres in diameter typically stimulate the growth of new blood vessels by secreting angiogenesis factors[21]. This 'neovascularisation' penetrates the lesion from its periphery and consists of thin-walled blood vessels that lack a muscular layer and often have chaotic anastomoses and arteriovenous shunts. High velocity flow results, especially in the feeding vessels, often with a disturbed (non-laminar) flow pattern that can be detected with Doppler as high velocity signals with a distinctive rasping sound. In addition, the anatomical display of colour Doppler allows a direct visualisation of the abnormal tumour vessels.

The Doppler effect is a phenomenon whereby the frequency of a wave received from a moving object is shifted relative to that of the original wave[22] (Fig. 1.5). When an ultrasound wave is transmitted into the tissue the frequency of the echoes from, for example, red blood cells moving towards the transducer is increased in proportion to their velocity, whereas red cells moving away from the transducer produce a fall in frequency. The frequency shift also depends on the original interrogating frequency and is affected by the angle between the beam and the direction of movement, only the component along the line of sight contributing to the shift, as indicated in the 'Doppler formula':

$$D = \pm \frac{2 f_0 \, V \cos \theta}{c}$$

where D is the Doppler shift frequency, f_0 is the frequency of the transmitted ultrasound beam via the blood velocity, c is the velocity of ultrasound in tissue and θ is the beam–vessel angle.

Since the cosine is zero when the angle between the beam and the blood flow is 90°, the Doppler shift becomes zero when the vessel runs directly across the beam and at this orientation no signal can be obtained. One of the main technical constraints with the clinical use of Doppler is optimising the beam–vessel angle, though the complex tangle of tumour vessels mitigates the problem in this particular situation.

The essence of extracting the Doppler shift signal consists of a comparison of the frequency of the transmitted and received waves. In order to facilitate this, either a continuous transmitted wave or, for pulsed systems, pulses longer than that for imaging are used. The electrical equivalents of the two are fed into comparator circuits which remove the signals from static interfaces and pass on the Doppler frequency shifts. Since various portions of the bloodstream in a real vessel are likely to be flowing at different velocities (depending on whether they are close to the vessel wall, for example), the resulting Doppler shifts cover a spectrum which can be extracted for display using a spectrum analyser (Fig. 1.6). By chance, the frequency shifts from blood fall into the audible range, and so can easily be output to a loudspeaker.

Doppler instruments are of three types: continuous wave, pulsed wave and colour flow.

Continuous wave doppler

Continuous wave (CW) Doppler instruments are the simplest type, consisting of a continuous wave voltage generator and a receiver/comparator circuit. The transducer is pencil-shaped and small and so can be applied directly to the skin. The sites of vessels can be traced using headphones or a video display and, if necessary, the characteristics of the blood flow can be displayed using a spectrum analyser. Continuous wave instruments detect flow anywhere within the overlapping region of the transmit and receive beams so that only crude depth information is available.

The early Doppler studies of the breast were performed with this type of system[20]. However, searching for small vessels with CW Doppler is time consuming, and comparison of mirror sites in the opposite breast was needed, so this technique was restricted to research studies.

Spectral (duplex) Doppler

If short bursts of ultrasound are transmitted into the patient, the delay in receipt of the echo indicates the depth of the vessel within the tissues just as with pulse-echo imaging. In pulsed Doppler only a selected region is sensitive and both its depth and length along the beam are under user control. Its position across the scan plane can also be selected. Thus the method allows specific regions in the real-time scan to be interrogated with detailed information about the presence and nature of blood flow extracted.

This type of pulsed Doppler is usually combined with real-time imaging (so-called duplex scanning), the position of the Doppler-sensitive gate being indicated on the real-time image. Because the pulses for imaging and Doppler are different (short for imaging, longer for Doppler), the scanner switches rapidly between the two modes, therefore less time can be spent in each mode and the frame rate for imaging and the pulse rate for Doppler are both reduced. In practice, for superficial structures the compromise is acceptable. As with CW Doppler, the signals are output either as a sound or as a spectral tracing. The great practical advantage of duplex systems is the simultaneous display of the blood flow spectrum and of the anatomy from which it derives.

Colour Doppler

The limitations of working with the small sensitive region in pulsed spectral Doppler have stimulated the development of systems that display blood flow over larger areas. One possibility is to employ multiple gates with parallel processing to extract multiple Doppler signals; not only is this exorbitantly expensive but, because the signal processing is slow, the resulting frame rate is unacceptably low. If, however, the entire train of echoes from one pulse is compared with those of a subsequent pulse (sent in exactly the same direction) by using an electronic device to cancel out the stationary echoes, then only signals from moving structures remain. This process is sufficiently fast for most purposes and produces a signal that is proportional to the mean Doppler shift together with an indication of the direction of flow.

The most useful way to display this data is as a colour-coded overlay upon the real-time gray-scale image[23] (Plate C.1). In practical terms, colour Doppler systems provide a moving picture of blood flow over the entire image area, allowing a rapid evaluation of tissue vascularity as well as providing a map for more detailed interroga-tion with spectral Doppler. The frame rate is reduced, but for small part applications such as the breast this is not disabling. There are limits to the low velocity and low volume flow sensitivity which mean that smaller normal and tumour vessels cannot be detected. Because, like all Doppler systems, colour Doppler is sensitive to all types of movement, unwanted signals due to breathing and transducer movements are suppressed by filters or, in more sophisticated systems, by intelligent motion dis-criminators.

Fig. 1.5
The Doppler effect
If an object moves toward the transducer (in practice, mainly blood cells in vessels), the frequency of the reflected ultrasound is higher than the transmitted frequency and vice versa for blood flowing away. This change of frequency is called the Doppler effect. The higher the velocity component in the direction of the transducer ($V \cos \theta$) and the higher the transmit frequency, the greater the frequency shift (Doppler shift).

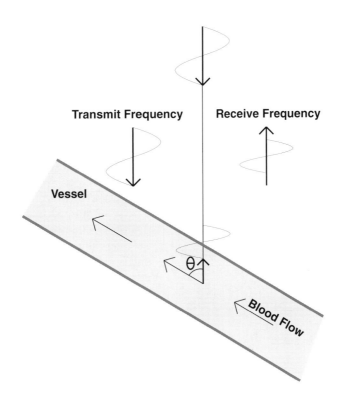

Fig. 1.6
The Doppler spectrum
The components of the Doppler shift signals are conventionally displayed as a spectrum on which the vertical axis indicates the Doppler shift frequency. (If the angle of the vessels can be determined, the true velocity of the blood flow can be derived but this is not always feasible for the small vessels in the breast since they may be too small to be visualised.) Signals above the baseline indicate flow towards the transducer while those below indicate flow away.
Pulsatile flow is typical of arteries and steady flow of veins. On this sonogram, signals from both an artery and vein are shown with flow in opposite directions. Veins may show pulsations in various situations, such as with arteriovenous fistula and because of transmission from an adjacent artery. Pulsation may also be seen in large veins, such as the axillary and subclavian veins, because of back flow from the heart.

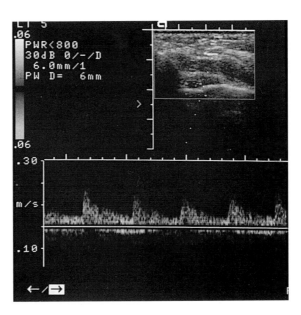

ARTEFACTS

Imaging artefacts

Central to ultrasound imaging is a series of assumptions about the behaviour of the ultrasound beam based on which the scanner constructs the images. The beam is considered to travel in a straight line, directly to and from the reflecting interface and at a constant velocity. The beam is also taken to be uniform and infinitely thin. Where these assumptions break down, artefacts are produced in the images. Understanding helps in the recognition and in avoiding misinterpretation of such artefacts.

Specular echoes – undetected surfaces

Where a flat surface is orientated at 90° to the ultrasound beam, echoes are received from it but, at other angles, the echoes tend to be directed away from the line of the transmitted beam and may not be detected. Theoretically, this means that truly flat surfaces orientated more than 20° away from normal are not detected, as can be demonstrated in water-tank experiments using glass or plastic plates. Fortunately, most tissue interfaces in the body in fact are a mixture of specular and scattering surfaces so that they usually do return echoes, even when orientated away from 90°. However, a surface that lies parallel to the ultrasound beam may not be visualised.

Slice thickness artefacts

The fact that the beam has a finite width means that reflectors lying to the side of the central beam axis can be detected by the scanner and displayed as though they lie on axis. The problem is more severe for strong reflectors which sometimes give falsely positioned echoes (e.g. at the periphery of cysts) (Fig. 1.7).

Reverberation artefacts

Echoes from an interface may be re-reflected from a second interface. Though usually these are not detected because they are weak and often do not return to the transducer, strong secondary reflections can give detectable signals and they are more obvious where the reflecting surfaces are flat and parallel to the skin, such as the anterior surface of a cyst. Here multiple reflections between two or more layers in or around the cyst wall may give repeated echoes that are displayed as parallel lines extending deep to the front surface (Fig. 1.8). The deeper echoes are progressively weakened because of attenuation in the tissue lying between the two surfaces. These 'reverberation artefacts' are particularly obvious in echo-free regions such as cysts because they stand out against the black background.

A similar effect may occur at the surface of gas bubbles, the sound reflecting between the bubbles but here producing a continuous stream of echoes because irregular fluid spaces between them produce effectively random path lengths. A bright streak, known as the 'comet tail artefact', is seen on the screen (e.g. from gas in a cyst that has been aspirated). Comet tails may also be seen deep to the surface of the lung (Fig. 1.9); this is more obvious after mastectomy, when the lung is closer to the skin.

Velocity artefacts

The assumption that the sound velocity in soft tissue is uniform is almost correct, there being little difference between sound speed in fat, glandular tissue, cyst fluid and solid lesions. However, the silicone material used in augmentation prostheses conducts ultrasound at only half the speed of soft tissue. Thus the ultrasound pulse takes twice as long to return so that the posterior surface of a prosthesis is depicted as lying twice as deep as it actually is (see Ch. 8.4).

Fig. 1.7
Slice thickness artefact (magnified image)
Low level echoes are depicted in the peripheral portions of the deeper cyst. This is because of the thickness of the ultrasound beam which falsely displays reflections from the cyst wall within the cavity. Note that they are not seen in the superficial cyst because this lies within the tightly focused part of the beam.

Gl: mammary gland

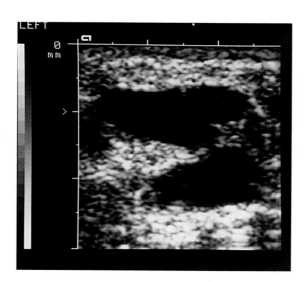

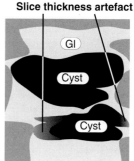

Slice thickness artefact

Gl

Cyst

Cyst

Fig. 1.8
Reverberation artefacts

When strong flat reflectors (interfaces) lie close together, a part of the reflected beam is re-reflected and returns a second time from the same interface. The multiple repeated reflections produce bands in the deeper parts of the breast (**a**). These repeated reflections are generally too weak to be apparent but may be obvious against a dark (poorly reflective) background especially in a cyst. In the scans in **b**, reverberations have occurred between the skin surface and the superficial layer of the superficial fascia. The reverberation artefacts in the subcutaneous fatty tissue are subtle (★) but those within the cysts are clearly seen. The clue to recognising this artefact is that the reverberations lie perpendicular to the ultrasound beam and parallel to each other, with a constant spacing. Since one of the interfaces is usually the transducer itself, use of a stand-off changes the spacing and alters or may suppress the reverberation.

SL: superficial layer of the superficial fascia

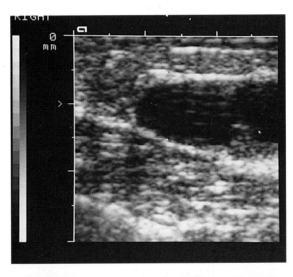

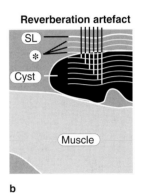

Reverberation artefact

b

Fig. 1.9
Reverberation artefacts

Air reflects almost all the incident ultrasound. Because the chest wall is thin after mastectomy, intense reverberation artefacts are commonly seen between the skin and the lung surface.

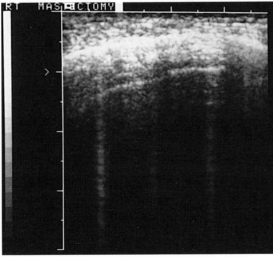

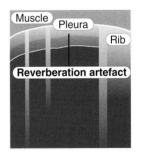

Shadowing and enhancement

Shadowing is the depiction of dark or black bands on the image due to reduced or absent sound transmission through an overlying object. Three types of acoustic shadowing may be recognised. Perhaps the most obvious is that produced by an interface which reflects most or all of the incident sound energy; such an interface is in effect 'opaque' to ultrasound and there is therefore less or no sound penetration to produce echoes from deeper-lying structures. This type of shadowing, *reflective shadowing*, is typically produced by gas and by extensive calcification. Tiny calcific foci (microcalcifications), though they may be extremely reflective and so produce strong echoes, are too small to interrupt enough of the sound beam to cause shadowing.

A second mechanism is *absorptive shadowing*. Ultrasound is progressively absorbed by being converted into heat in soft tissues. The average loss of sound by this means is corrected for by progressive increase in amplification, adjusted by the TGC control. However, if a region of tissue, (e.g. a fibrotic area) attenuates more strongly than the average, then less sound will penetrate, resulting in a partial shadow. Attenuative shadowing is a typical feature of breast carcinomas where it is proportional to the amount of fibrous stroma in the lesion. It is also seen behind operative scars.

A third mechanism of shadowing is *edge or interface shadowing*; this is seen as fine, dark lines extending deep from oblique flat or curved surfaces such as Cooper's ligaments or the edges of masses (Fig. 1.10). The underlying mechanism of these edge or 'lateral shadows' is complex and probably involves a combination of absorption and refraction. Since they have no diagnostic significance, it is important that they are not confused with the broader shadows due to absorption or reflection.

The reverse of attenuation shadowing is *acoustic enhancement*. Here a bright band extends beyond the enhancing structure, the effect being due to a region with less attenuation than the surrounding tissue for which the TGC is set to compensate. It is typically produced by fluid-containing structures such as cysts and also by solid tissues with a high water content, such as fibroadenomas and phylloides tumours.

Fig. 1.10
Edge (interface) shadowing
Narrow bands of shadowing fall deep to the curved surface at the lateral border of this fibroadenoma. Known as 'edge shadows', they do not have the same suspicious significance as attenuative shadowing, being typical of benign lesions. The mechanism of this type of shadowing is probably a mixture of absorption and refraction (beam spreading).

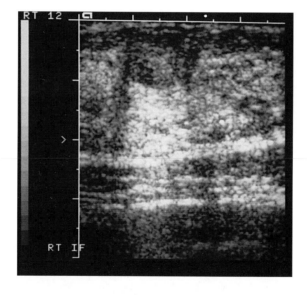

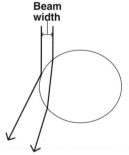

Beam width

Doppler artefacts

Aliasing

Aliasing is the most important Doppler artefact. It is the erroneous depiction of flow velocity and direction that arises because the rate at which the moving blood is being sampled (i.e. the pulse repetition frequency, PRF) is too slow to allow an accurate reconstruction of the true velocity. Any manoeuvre that reduces the Doppler frequency shift can be used to minimise or eliminate aliasing; increasing the interrogation angle or using a lower frequency transducer are examples. Similarly, any manoeuvre that increases the PRF is effective; the usual way to achieve this is to increase the frequency (velocity) scale, which is internally linked to the PRF. Since the PRF is limited by the depth of tissue to be interrogated, aliasing is less marked for superficial vessels and in practice is not a major problem in breast Doppler.

On the spectral trace the phenomenon is seen as a truncation of the highest velocity traces at one limit of the scale, the aliased signal appearing in the opposite direction (Fig. 1.11). It may be re-located by shifting the position of the zero baseline. In colour Doppler the aliased signals appear as regions with an abrupt transition between fast forward and fast reverse flow (or vice versa) giving a mosaic pattern to the image (Plate C.2). This is in contra-distinction to true flow reversal in which the blood is always stationary for a short period of time and thus gives a zero signal that appears as black borders to the colour signals.

Fig. 1.11
Aliasing on Doppler
High velocity signals are displayed as flow in the reverse direction (arrows in **a**). This erroneous depiction of the flow velocity is caused by the ultrasound pulse rate (pulse repetition frequency, PRF) being too slow to sample the fast blood flow adequately. The artefact is most readily removed by increasing the scale to display higher velocity flow (this automatically increases the PRF) (**b**), or by changing the angle of the Doppler beam to reduce cosine θ.

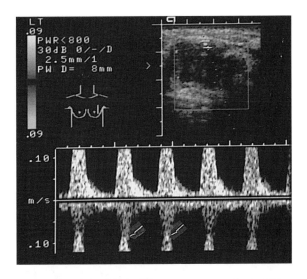

a

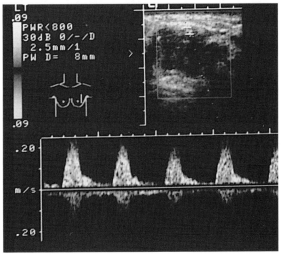

b

Mirror signals

In some situations signals are seen simultaneously on both sides of the baseline of the spectral trace, implying simultaneous forward and reverse flow within the Doppler range gate (Fig. 1.12). This may be a true depiction of the blood flow: for example, where there are two vessels lying close together, where the vasculature is tortuous (as in tumour vessels) or where there is flow disturbance producing vortices with true flow reversal. In these situations the shapes of the forward and reverse spectra are almost always slightly different from each other. A similar appearance may be artefactual, most commonly occurring when the Doppler gain is set too high so that the Doppler circuitry is overloaded and fails to discriminate properly between forward and reverse flow. A similar effect may be produced when a vessel is interrogated in cross-section and at 90° to the blood flow; here the Doppler shift is extremely low and minor variations with pulsation or due to streaming within the vessel may produce signals in both directions. In this case the pattern is seen to be unstable with time on the spectral trace.

Another mechanism that can produce a similar effect occurs with wide aperture transducers; for a vessel lying close to the transducer and at a large θ angle, elements at one end may truly detect blood flowing towards the transducer at the same time as elements from the other end detect blood flowing away from it. In both these cases the two signals have the same configuration, although sometimes one is more intense that the other.

With colour Doppler the mirror artefact is not usually apparent because the computer logic is set to display the fastest flow at any given pixel on the reasonable assumption that blood cannot be flowing in two directions simultaneously in one location. However, a different type of mirror artefact is sometimes encountered with colour Doppler whereby a second vessel with identical anatomical and flow properties is seen apparently across a strongly reflecting surface such as the lung. This is produced by the air surface acting as a true acoustic mirror, resulting in a mirror image, just as may occur with grey-scale imaging (Plate C.3).

Fig. 1.12

Mirror spectral Doppler artefact

The Doppler spectrum is displayed on both sides of the baseline as though reflected in a mirror (**a**). There are several varieties of this phenomenon: (1) Two vessels of opposite direction may lie in the sample volume, as often happens with the tortuous vessels typical of tumours. In this case the velocity and phase are unlikely to be identical for the different vessels, so the 'mirror' tracing is not identical to the main spectrum. (2) If the flow is perpendicular to the ultrasound beam, some flow is detected as flow towards the transducer and some as away because of the beam width. This geometric arrangement gives poor signals with noise and low Doppler shift frequencies. (3) The commonest cause is excessive Doppler gain, so that the Doppler circuits are overloaded and fail to discriminate the direction properly. In this case the spectral gray-scale is saturated to a complete white and the mirror signals disappear on reducing the Doppler gain (**b**).

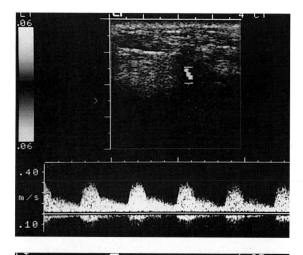

a

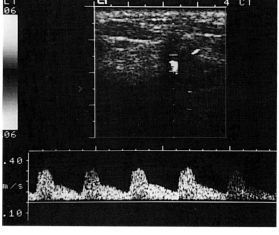

b

BIOLOGICAL EFFECTS OF ULTRASOUND

Ultrasound interacts with biological tissue in two main ways: thermal and non-thermal. Thermal interaction entails the conversion of ultrasound energy into heat due to absorption in the tissues. For diagnostic ultrasound thermal effects are minimal even in non-perfused tissues, and where there is a blood supply the heat is rapidly dissipated. Non-thermal effects are more complex and not fully understood. The most important are cavitation and interaction with gas bubbles. If the decompression phase of the ultrasound pulse is sufficiently intense, microbubbles of gas are formed in the tissue. These and any spontaneously occurring bubbles can be stimulated to grow by the incident ultrasound energy if they are of a size comparable to the wavelength. In this case they vibrate violently and are capable of disrupting cell membranes. Cavitation and bubble effects only develop under continuous insonation and thus are unlikely to occur with the short pulses used in ultrasound imaging. There is a slightly greater risk with the longer pulses used in Doppler and most particularly with ultrasound therapy.

Ultrasound intensity is measured as the energy flowing across a surface, in units of watts per centimetre squared (W/cm^2). For pulsed ultrasound, the peak values, which are more relevant to cavitation effects, may be used, but averages over the duration of the pulse sequence are considered to give a truer representation of the absorbed dose, relevant to thermal effects. Due to focusing, the spatial peak intensity is usually quoted. At the frequencies used for ultrasound diagnosis there have been no independently confirmed significant biological effects in mammalian tissues exposed in vivo to intensities (spatial peak temporal average) measured in a free field of water below 100 mW/cm^2 and this is recommended by the American Institute of Ultrasound in Medicine as the maximum level suitable for diagnostic use[24]. It should be noted, however, that even at much higher intensities no significant effects have been consistently demonstrated provided the exposure times are reasonably short. In fact, tissue absorption allows for higher intensities than those measured in a water-bath, so that these figures can be doubled in practice whilst still remaining within safe limits for the tissues actually being examined. While the intensities from most scanners are within these limits, those for some arrays are on the high side and these rise markedly when they are operated in the spectral (pulsed) Doppler mode though less so in colour Doppler.

REFERENCES

1. J.J. Wild, J.M. Reid: Further pilot echographic studies on the histologic structure of tumors of the living intact human breast. Am J Pathol 28; 839–861, 1952.
2. D.H. Howry, D.A. Stott, W.R. Bliss: The ultrasonic visualization of carcinoma of the breast and other soft-tissue structures. Cancer 7; 354–358, 1954.
3. G. Kossoff, J. Jellins: The physics of breast echography. Seminars in Ultrasound 3; 5–12, 1982.
4. L.W. Bassett, R.H. Gold, C. Kimme-Smith: Hand-Held and Automated Breast Ultrasound. Slack, New Jersey, 1986.
5. P.J. Dempsey, M. Moskowitz: Is there a role for breast sonography? In: Controversies in Ultrasound —Clinics of Diagnostic Ultrasound (20), edited by J.P. McGahan. Churchill Livingstone, New York, 1987, pp17–36.
6. Y. Kikuchi, R. Uchida, K. Tanaka, T. Wagai: Early cancer diagnosis through ultrasonics. J Acoust Soc Am 29; 824–833, 1957.
7. E. Kelly-Fry: Breast imaging. In: Ultrasound Applied to Obstetrics and Gynecology, edited by R.E. Sabbagha. Harper & Row, New York, 1980, pp 327–350.
8. J. Jellins, T.S. Reeve, J. Croll, G. Kossoff: Results of breast echography examination in Sydney, Australia 1972–1979. In: Seminars in Ultrasound, edited by H.W. Raymond and W.J. Zwiebel. Grune & Stratton, New York, 1982, pp 58–62.
9. J. Jellins, G. Kossoff, F.W. Buddee, T.S. Reeve: Ultrasonic visualisation of the breast. Med J Aust 1; 305–307, 1971.
10. E. Kelly-Fry: Influence on the development of ultrasound pulse-echo breast instrumentation in the United States. In: Ultrasound Mammography, edited by P. Harper. University Park Press, Baltimore, 1985.
11. F.H. DeLand: A modified technique of ultrasonography for the detection and differential diagnosis of breast lesions. AJR 105; 446–452, 1969.
12. T. Wagai, M. Tsutsumi: Ultrasound examination of the breast. In: Breast Carcinoma: The Radiologist's Expanded Role, edited by W.W. Logan. Wiley, New York, 1977, pp 325–342.
13. G. Kossoff, D.A. Carpenter, D.E. Robinson, et al: Octoson—a new rapid general purpose echoscope. In: Ultrasound in Medicine, Vol. 2, edited by D. White, R. Barnes. Plenum Press, New York, 1976, p 333.
14. F.S. Foster, M. Arditi, M.S. Patterson, et al: Breast imaging with a conical transducer/annular array hybrid scanner. Ultrasound Med Biol 9; 151–164, 1983.
15. G. Baum: Ultrasound mammography. Radiology 122; 199–205, 1977.
16. S.v.W. Hilton, G.R. Leopold, L.K. Olson, S.A. Willson: Real-time breast sonography: application in 300 consecutive patients. AJR 147; 479–486, 1986.
17. L.W. Bassett, C. Kimme-Smith, L.K. Sutherland, et al: Automated and hand-held breast US: effect on patient management. Radiology 165; 103–108, 1987.
18. M.M. Vilaro, A.B. Kurtz, L. Needleman, et al: Hand-held and automated sonomammography: clinical role relative to X-ray mammography. J Ultrasound Med 8; 95–100,1989.
19. E. Goldman: The growth of malignant disease in man and the lower animals with special reference to the vascular system. Proc R Soc Med 1; 3, 1902.
20. P.N. Burns, J.D. Davies, M. Halliwell, et al: Doppler ultrasound in the diagnosis of breast cancer. In: Ultrasound in Breast and Endocrine Disease—Clinics in Diagnostic Ultrasound (12), edited by G.R. Leopold. Churchill Livingstone, New York, 1984, pp 41–56.
21. A.M. Schor, S.L. Schor: Tumour angiogenesis. J Pathol 141: 385–413, 1983.
22. P.N.T. Wells: Basic principles and Doppler physics. In: Clinical Applications of Doppler Ultrasound, edited by K.J.W. Taylor, P.N. Burns, P.N.T. Wells. Raven Press, New York, 1988, pp 1–25.
23. D.O. Cosgrove, J.C. Bamber, J.B. Davey et al: Colour Doppler signals from breast tumours, work in progress. Radiology 176; 175–180, 1990.
24. American Institute of Ultrasound in Medicine: Bioeffects Considerations for the Safety of Diagnostic Ultrasound. American Institute of Ultrasound in Medicine, Bethesda, MD, 1988.

Chapter 2

Scanning techniques

PATIENT POSITION

With a real-time scanner, the ultrasound examination of the breast can be performed with the patient in any position as necessitated by her condition. However, the use of a standard position and uniform technique facilitates subsequent analysis of the scans and improves reproducibility as well as localisation of lesions. After palpation of both breasts to locate any obvious abnormality, the patient is asked to lie supine and turn slightly to the contralateral side with the ipsilateral arm raised over her head; a pillow placed under the shoulder of the side to be examined makes this more comfortable. This posture flattens the breast onto the chest wall and positions it symmetrically

and reproducibly; it also facilitates examining the inferior portion of the breast and the axilla. For large breasts, placing the arm down to stretch the skin folds makes examination of the upper part of the breast easier. For the same reason, a more oblique posture is preferable for the lateral part and a supine position for the medial part.

If intracystic echoes such as a fluid–fluid or fat–fluid level are suspected on the initial scan, asking to the patient to turn over or sit up while observing postural changes in the level is often helpful in discriminating these complex cavities from artefacts or true solid structures (Fig. 2.1).

Fig. 2.1
Fat–fluid level—changes with patient positioning
This postoperative cyst contains a small amount of fat which is seen as an echogenic crescent close to the transducer, floating above the serous component (**a**). After moving the patient to the sitting position, the longitudinal scan shows that the fat–fluid level has shifted to remain horizontal (**b**). The echoes behind the fluid are enhanced, but those behind the fat are attenuated (shadowing).

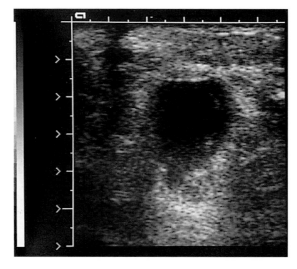

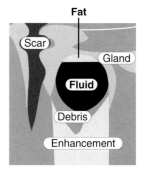

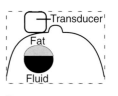

a

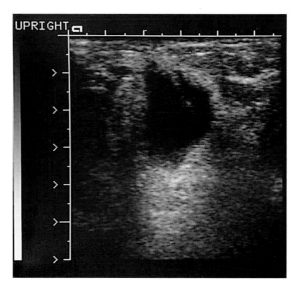

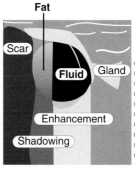

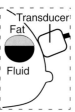

b

SCANNING TECHNIQUE

After spreading acoustic coupling gel on to the skin, scanning may be initiated in any direction (e.g. transversely, longitudinally or radially—when the transducer is rotated around the nipple). Whatever method is adopted, it is essential that the entire breast, including the axillary tail, is examined systematically. In the involuted breast, glandular tissue only remains in the central portion because it is first replaced by fat and connective tissues in the peripheral portions; however, a carcinoma may develop in residual ducts apparently remote from the demonstrable gland, so the scan must cover the entire breast, not just the persisting glandular portion. The region to be scanned extends from the clavicle down to below the inframammary fold (the mammary gland may even extend slightly below the inframammary fold), and from the sternal border medially to the midaxillary line laterally. If a lesion is detected, it is important that it be imaged from many directions to ensure that the findings are reproducible and to evaluate its overall appearances and relationships with surrounding tissues. Intraductal lesions and the relationships of a mass to the ducts are best demonstrated by radial scanning or scanning along the ducts.

Superficial lesions may be more clearly visualised by using a stand-off to place the lesion at the best focal region and reduce superimposed reverberation artefacts. Several stand-offs are available commercially (e.g. Kitecko® (3M), Aquaflex® (Parker Laboratories) or Sonar-Aid® (Geistlich)). They are convenient in use because of their physical consistency and acoustic characteristics but, if these are unavailable, a water-bag or a thick layer of contact gel form an effective substitute.

When a palpable abnormality is demonstrated, holding the lesion with the free hand during scanning confirms that the image corresponds with the mass. Without simultaneous palpation, isoechoic lesions (i.e. those with the same reflectivity as the background) may be missed entirely, while encapsulated fat or thickened but normal glandular tissues may cause a palpable 'abnormality' that can readily be correlated with the ultrasound image.

Portions of the fatty tissue of the breast sometimes become intermingled with the glandular tissue; known as 'fat islands', they may mimic an echo-poor intraglandular lesion. Actually, most are in continuity with the subcutaneous fat, so that they would be better described as 'peninsulas' than as islands. Demonstrating continuity of the fat island with the surrounding fatty tissue (by scanning from various angles and rotating the transducer) and ascertaining that its internal texture is the same as that of the fatty tissue helps avoid misdiagnosis (Fig. 2.2). Like fat islands, fatty tissue in general is very soft and easily compressible under probe compression (see section on 'dynamic tests' in this chapter).*

LABELLING

A clock-face is used to indicate the location of images or the site of lesions. If distance from the nipple is important (e.g. for locating a mass), this can be added as a second numeral in centimetres (Fig. 2.4).

---

* **Note**: Side-by-side, 'dual', images. To compensate for the small field of view provided by linear array transducers, some of the images in this book are presented as a pair of two adjacent scans, known as 'dual imaging' (Fig. 2.3). Artificial dark lines at the centre of the composite image mark the junction between the two components.

Fig. 2.2
Fat island

An echo-poor area in the mammary gland simulates an intraglandular lesion (**a**) but, by rotating the transducer, this 'lesion' can be seen to be continuous with the subcutaneous layer, demonstrating that it is part of the fatty tissue (**b**). Two other fat islands are also seen in **b**. On dynamic compression, fat islands are readily compressible, unlike fibroadenomas, which they may resemble on the scan.

Gl: mammary gland
SCF: subcutaneous fat

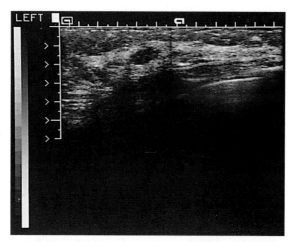

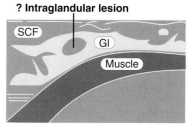

a

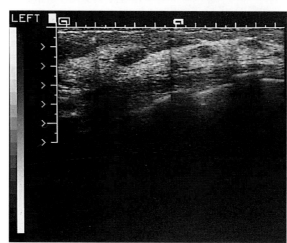

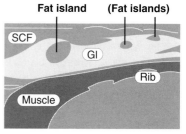

b

Fig. 2.3
Side-by-side (dual) image
The width of the linear array used for
this scan is 3.8 cm so the 2 cm
fibroadenoma shown occupies almost
the entire field of view (**a**). By
combining two images in a composite
'dual' scan (**b**), the relation between
the fibroadenoma and the surrounding
glandular tissue is better displayed.
The dark line depicted in the centre of
the image is an artefact that
represents the edges of the
contiguous scans. Because the two
components are aligned manually,
there may be overlap or a gap
between the two portions; therefore,
measurements should not be made
across the join line.

Fa: fibroadenoma
Gl: mammary gland
ES: edge shadow
PE: posterior enhancement

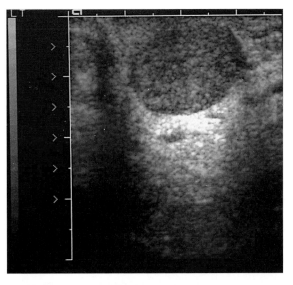

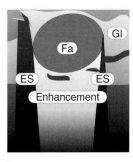

a

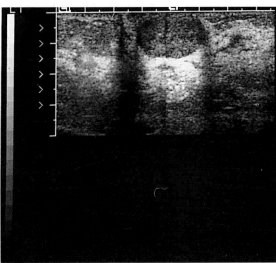

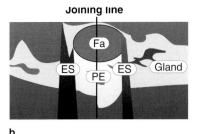

b

Fig. 2.4
Labelling
This lesion in the upper inner quadrant
of the right breast is described as Rt.
(2,3), i.e. it lies at the 2 o'clock position
in the right breast and is 3 cm away
from the nipple.

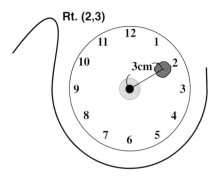

MEASUREMENT OF TUMOUR SIZE

Although clinically the measurement of the largest palpable axis is commonly quoted as the size of a mass, with ultrasound all three dimensions, the transverse and longitudinal diameters and the depth can be measured and the tumour volume calculated if needed. Size assessed on ultrasound correlates well with histological measurements[1], though both are usually smaller than that measured on palpation. There are two reasons for this: (1) on palpation the thickness of the surrounding tissue is also included, a discrepancy that is exaggerated when the lesion is deeply situated; (2) in invasive lesions, the surrounding tissues which are oedematous, or have undergone reactive desmoplastic changes microscopically, are firm on palpation whereas on ultrasound the outer limits of these changes are difficult to visualise. This discrepancy is particularly marked with carcinomas and is also recognised when comparing palpation with X-ray mammography where it is known as Le Borgne's Law. For lesions with a halo or boundary echoes (see Ch. 4), measurements that include the halo best reflect the true size of the tumour when related to histology (Fig. 2.5), although the outer limit is often difficult to determine precisely because it is ill-defined, as is typical of the scirrhous type of carcinoma. For follow-up of changes in tumour size, measurements of the nidus may be more useful because they are more reproducible, especially on frozen images.

The volume of a lesion is calculated on the assumption that it approximates an ovoid in shape:

$$V\,(\mathrm{cm}^3) = (D_1 \times D_2 \times D_3) / 2$$

where D_1 = transverse diameter (cm), D_2 = longitudinal diameter (cm), and D_3 = depth (cm).

DYNAMIC TESTS

Observing the compressibility of a lesion and its mobility within the surrounding tissue with a real-time scanner gives useful additional information about the nature of a lesion. The simplest method is to compress the lesion directly with the transducer and evaluate its consistency by comparing its movements with those of the surrounding soft breast tissues; alternatively, the lesion can be compressed from the sides between the fingers of the free hand, and this is often a more sensitive method of demonstrating compressibility. In the same way, mobility can be demonstrated by attempting to twist or rotate the lesion while observing its movements in real-time (Figs 2.6–2.8). Lesions that are locally fixed tend to drag the surrounding tissues with them as they move, whereas freely mobile lesions, notably fibroadenomas, slip through the tissues without disturbing them.

Fig. 2.5
Measurement of tumour size
The echogenic halo should be included in the measurement of a carcinoma because it represents the growing edge of the tumour. Since the halo is not always clear, especially on frozen images, the size of the nidus may have to be measured, especially for serial studies. For tumours with strong shadowing, as in this case, the deep margin of the tumour is not seen so measurement of the AP diameter is difficult.

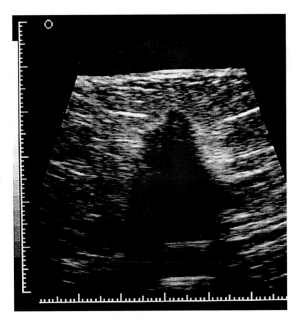
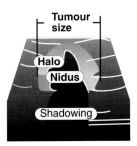

Fig. 2.6
Dynamic tests
The most sensitive way to visualise the compressibility of a mass is to grip the lesion with the free hand and compress it from the sides while observing the response on real-time (straight arrows). Mobility is best evaluated by attempting to twist the lesion in the same way (curved arrows).

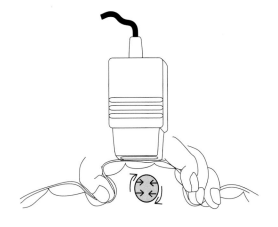

Fig. 2.7
Compressibility
This lesion has low level internal echoes and only slight posterior enhancement (i.e. it is a complex cyst, see Chapter 6.1) (**a**). However, it is easily deformed by compression from the sides (**b**), making malignancy unlikely.

DL: deep layer of the superficial fascia
IS: interface shadow from Cooper's ligament
RMS: retromammary space
SL: superficial layer of the superficial fascia.
SCF: subcutaneous fat

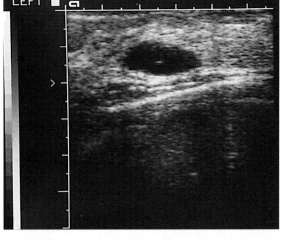

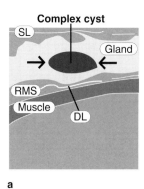

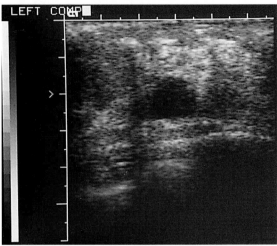

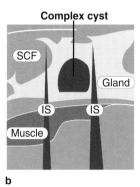

Fig. 2.8
Mobility
This slightly lobulated echo-poor mass has well-defined margins and posterior enhancement—the classical appearances of a fibroadenoma (**a**). Twisting the lesion with the free hand causes it to rotate through 90° (**b**); such mobility is typical of a fibroadenoma .

ES: edge shadow
Fa: fibroadenoma
PE: posterior enhancement

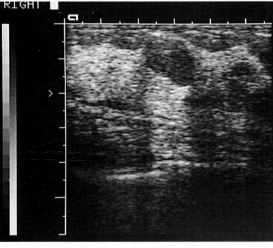

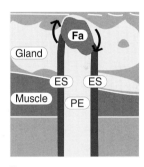

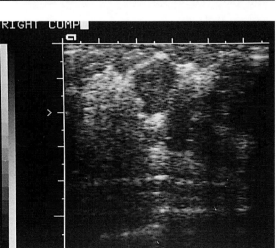

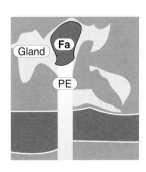

LYMPH NODES

If malignancy is suspected, a search for lymph node metastases is important for staging and management. Both the axillary and internal mammary lymph node areas should be checked; ultrasound evaluation of the latter is especially important because nodes here are impalpable.

The axillary region can be examined by sweeping the transducer downwards from the apex of the axilla on the chest wall along the lateral margin of the pectoralis major muscle. The soft axillary lymph nodes that are often normally palpable and are readily demonstrated on X-ray mammograms are difficult to detect on ultrasound because their fat content gives them the same appearances as the surrounding axillary fat. Pathological lymph nodes, however, are readily visualised on ultrasound.

Internal mammary lymph nodes are best detected on longitudinal scans sweeping laterally from the edge of the sternum for several centimetres. They lie within the intercostal spaces, so that the shadowing that may be produced by the costal cartilages when they are calcified is not a practical limitation. The first, second, third and fourth intercostal spaces should be examined carefully since most nodes lie at this level.

In advanced malignancy, longitudinal scans along the axillary and subclavian vessels may reveal level II or III axillary lymphadenopathy (deep to and medial to pectoralis minor muscle, respectively) as well as the interpectoral (Rotter) nodes lying near the origin of the thoraco-acromial vessels.

DOPPLER

Using a CW Doppler flowmeter, the sites of strong vascular signals can be located and traced out using a pencil transducer. This technique is too time consuming to be practical for routine use. With duplex scanners, which combine a real-time imaging scanner with a Doppler system, the lesion and the surrounding tissues can be examined with slow searches. This technique is also tedious because the tumour or feeding vessels are usually too small to be visualised on the B-mode images. By combing real-time imaging with colour flow mapping (generally known as 'colour Doppler') the Doppler examination can be performed much more quickly and easily so that it is feasible to include Doppler as a part of the routine study. The thorough search that is possible with colour Doppler lends much more confidence in a negative study where no flow can be demonstrated. Information about the vascular anatomy is also obtained, including the number of vessels and their arrangement and configuration (straight or tangled), as well as the anatomical relationships between the vessels and the lesion.

For a Doppler examination minimal pressure of the transducer must be used to avoid compressing low pressure vessels. Starting with settings optimised to detect weak and low velocity signals (highest frequency transducer; minimum filter and grey/colour thresholding; lowest maximum velocity range; gain set at a level where colour noise just disappears), slow searches sweeping through the region of interest are used. Changing the interrogation angle helps detect blood flowing parallel to the skin which otherwise fails to give a Doppler shift signal because there is no flow component in the direction of the beam. Reducing the colour mapping area (especially the width) increases the frame rate*. Signals from vessels can be recognised by their pulsating and anatomically constant nature compared with the randomly varying signals from noise. The velocity range may need to be adjusted to avoid aliasing. The vascular density (the number of vessels) and their relations with a lesion (e.g. feeding artery, draining vein or simply a normal adjacent vessel) can be evaluated on colour Doppler. As Doppler systems have improved in sensitivity, more normal vessels in the breast have become detectable, so the differentiation between them and pathological vessels has become more difficult. Their typical positions (along the glandular surface or running with the Cooper's ligaments) and the straight or gently curved path of normal vessels are helpful in their distinction from pathological vessels which tend to be numerous, tortuous and abnormally positioned. Comparison with the contralateral breast or quantitative studies may also be helpful.

Spectral analysis confirms that the colour signals are truly from a vessel and help determine the type of vessel, whether artery or vein. For spectral analysis, the sensitive gate is placed on the vessel detected on colour Doppler. As with colour Doppler, the threshold for velocity and gain are initially set at maximum sensitivity. Once Doppler signals are obtained, the velocity scale may need adjustment to display the highest velocities without aliasing and the gain should be adjusted to display the spectral waveform as a grey-scale. The angle of the Doppler beam may also need to be changed. In the breast the blood vessels themselves are usually too small to be imaged, so the beam–vessel angle correction is difficult to set accurately and true velocity measurements cannot be made; this difficulty can sometimes be circumvented if colour Doppler is available. However, the pulsatility index (PI) or resistance index (RI) can be used to quantify the circulatory resistance of the arterioles beyond the measurement point because these ratios are not angle dependent (Fig. 2.9). Tumour vessels usually have a low resistance to flow but the value of the indices in the differential diagnosis of breast lesions has not been determined.

INTERVENTIONAL TECHNIQUES

The use of ultrasound to guide needling is now a widely accepted technique[2]. Fine needle aspiration to evacuate cysts and for cytological diagnosis and localisation before biopsy are the main purposes of the ultrasound guided interventional procedures for the breast[3-6]. Cutting biopsies for histology are occasionally indicated.

Fine needle aspiration cytology

Fine needle aspiration cytology (FNAC) is widely used for breast lesions and improves diagnostic accuracy[7].

---

* Colour Capture. All the colour Doppler images in this book were taken in the 'colour capture' mode (Plate C.4). This stores and displays the highest value signal at each location over a preset time (4 s is usually used), during which the transducer is slowly rocked through the region of interest. Colour capture images more closely represent the impression gained during the real-time colour Doppler scan because the three-dimensional network of vessels is better represented and, for arteries, the flow in systole is displayed.

Cytological preparations differ from histological sections in that the aspirated cells are dispersed and so the architectural features are usually lost. The main thrust of cytological interpretation is the distinction between benign and malignant cells without further characterisation of the lesion from which they were aspirated. Five categories of cytological opinion are used by most laboratories: C0 = unsatisfactory specimen (scanty or poorly cellular sample or cellular sample with preparation artefacts); C1 = benign (Plate P.2.1); C2 = probably benign; C3 = equivocal; C4 = suspicious, probably malignant; C5 = malignant (Plate P.2.2).

False positive cytological diagnoses of malignancy should be very rare, but in practice reach 0.5%. False negative diagnoses are determined by diverse factors such as the accuracy of localisation of the lesion with the needle, preparative artefacts and difficulties with cytological interpretation, but should be less than 10% on satisfactory smears taken from palpable lesions.

The wide use of ultrasound and X-ray mammography reveals many non-palpable lesions whose nature cannot always be determined on the images alone. FNAC is more easily guided by ultrasound than by X-ray mammography because the tip of the needle can be followed throughout the procedure in real-time. X-ray mammographically guided FNAC is required for lesions that are undetectable on ultrasound, preferably using stereotactic methods to locate the lesion and the tip of the needle in three dimensions[8,9]. The indications for FNAC are wide because it is minimally invasive. Generally they are as follows:

1. Non-palpable breast lesions whose nature cannot be determined by imaging. In practice, asymptomatic simple cysts are excluded because their diagnosis is certain on ultrasound. Breast carcinomas, especially the well-circumscribed type, may have a very similar appearance to benign lesions, so all solid lesions as well as complex cysts, particularly in women over middle age, need further evaluation by cytology and/or follow-up. Fluid aspirated from cysts need not be sent for cytological examination unless it is blood-stained or if the cyst is recurrent or if a mass persists after aspiration.

2. Vaguely palpable or palpable but small or deep lesions. A mass behind the breast originating from the chest wall muscles or the pleural cavity may present as a breast tumour. Clinically guided cytology in these cases is often negative because they lie deeper than they seem on palpation. FNAC under ultrasound guidance, or a planning ultrasound scan to determine the depth of the lesion, is recommended.

3. Intracystic tumours. Cytological sampling of the solid part is needed for correct diagnosis and this requires ultrasound guidance.

4. Lesions close to an implant to avoid puncture of the implant.

Almost the only complication is haematoma which can be avoided by adequate compression after needle withdrawal and rarely needs treatment. Pneumothorax, a recognised complication of needling under palpation, has not been reported when ultrasound is used for guidance. Needle-track seeding of carcinoma has never been reported in the breast after needle cytology or tumour localisation[10–12]. There are no contraindications to this fine needle method except lack of patient cooperation.

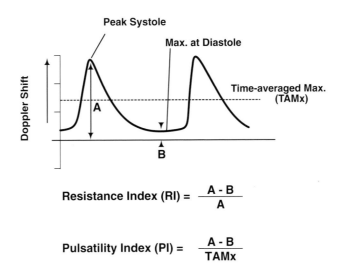

Fig. 2.9
Resistance index (RI) and pulsatility index (PI)
The resistance and pulsatility indices are useful to evaluate the resistance to flow of the arteriolar bed. These indices are angle independent. RI and PI are usually low in tumour vessels.

$$\text{Resistance Index (RI)} = \frac{A - B}{A}$$

$$\text{Pulsatility Index (PI)} = \frac{A - B}{TAMx}$$

Methods

There are two general methods, either freehand or using a guidance system. The choice depends on the experience of the examiner though a needle guidance system is generally simpler for beginners and is preferred in large, deformable breasts; however, needle guides are not available for all transducers. If the guidance system necessitates a change to a transducer that gives less good images, the losses may outweigh the benefits. A detachable adaptor is a good compromise if the scanner is equipped to indicate the needle path as an overlay on the image.

Freehand technique (Fig. 2.10)

The patient is placed in the same position as for scanning. The skin is cleaned with a sterilising solution and the gel-coated transducer is wrapped in a plastic film (e.g. domestic cling film) for cleanliness and to avoid damage to its surface by the sterilising solution. Strict sterilisation of the transducer (e.g. with ethylene oxide gas) is not necessary for this minimally invasive technique. Heat sterilisation should never be used because it is almost certain to damage the transducer. Some transducers can be sterilised in antiseptic solutions; the manufacturer's advice should be sought.

After sterilised gel has been spread onto the skin, the transducer is placed over the lesion at a suitable site for puncture. The areolar and nipple regions should be avoided because these areas are very sensitive and the skin and connective tissues are thicker. The optimum angle for insertion is about 45° but tends to be more for deep lesions (to shorten the distance) and less for superficial lesions (to allow imaging of a reasonable length of the needle). Local anaesthesia is not required because the needle is thin, though some patients strongly request it.

For aspiration a 25 mm, 23-gauge, standard venepuncture needle is generally satisfactory, with a 10 ml disposable syringe attached; the needle selected depends on the depth and appearances of the lesion. For example, if a cyst with inspissated material is suspected, a thicker needle is likely to be needed to evacuate the viscid contents.

The needle is visualised as a bright line on the image and its position can be confirmed by to-and-fro movements (Fig. 2.11). Once the tip of the needle has been positioned in the lesion, the syringe plunger is withdrawn to apply a vacuum. During aspiration the needle is moved to-and-fro and rotated in the lesion to ensure adequate sampling. If maintaining suction with one hand is difficult, a special device attached to the syringe may be useful, though these make the syringe heavy and are clumsy, impairing precise insertion under ultrasound guidance. An alternative is to attach the syringe to the needle by an extension tube and ask an assistant to withdraw the plunger. After releasing the vacuum (the plunger should be freed but not pushed back as this may eject the specimen), the needle is withdrawn.

The aspirated material is smeared thinly on microscope slides. Because the aspirate is usually scanty and may remain within the barrel of the needle, the syringe should be detached from the needle, filled with air and reattached to the needle before the aspirate is ejected forcibly. The slides are dried rapidly in air (a hair dryer may be used) for Giemsa staining or fixed with spirit for Papanicolaou staining. Preparation in both ways is rec-ommended when more than two slides are available, the thinner one being preferred for Giemsa staining.

FNAC with a needle guide system

After cleaning or draping the transducer (the method depends on the transducer, as described above), the sterilised guide is attached. Longer needles, such as those used for spinal puncture or PTC (percutaneous transhepatic cholangiography), are required for this system (Fig. 2.12). The path of the needle is usually displayed as an electronically generated overlay on the screen and the transducer is positioned so that the guide line crosses the centre of the lesion. With this system, aspiration is more easily performed by two people, the operator holding the transducer and steadying the breast while the needle is inserted by the assistant. The ease of aspiration using a needle guide depends on how clearly the tip of the needle is visualised on the image. Because choosing or changing the angle after skin puncture is difficult with a needle guide, the freehand technique is more flexible.

Fig. 2.10
Freehand ultrasound needle guidance
The freehand technique is the simplest method of needle guidance under ultrasound. The transducer must be positioned to show both the needle and the lesion simultaneously.

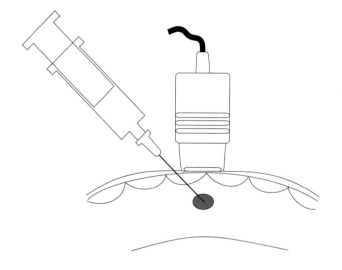

Fig. 2.11
Aspiration cytology under ultrasound guidance
The needle is clearly seen as an echogenic line with its tip in the echo-poor lesion. Because both ultrasound appearances and the cytology were benign, this lesion was not excised but was followed clinically.

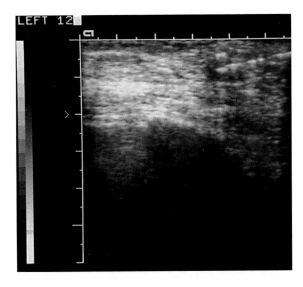

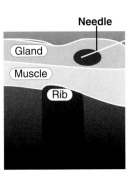

Fig. 2.12
Adapter for needle insertion
A detachable adapter forms a convenient and precise needle guide. A longer needle is required for this procedure (Aloka).

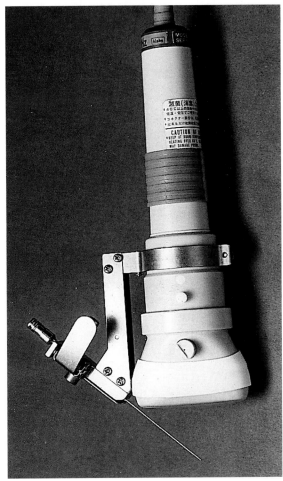

Localisation

The technique of needle insertion is almost the same as that for an aspiration. Several types of the localisation needle are available, including a hookwire (DKBL Breast Lesion Localizer, Cook Inc., Bloomington, IN)[13], a curved-end retractable wire (Mammo-Lock)[14] or one of the retractable-barb needles (Reidy-X, Cook Inc., Bloomington, IN; N.S. Medical Products, Gainesville, FA)[15]. Because the 20-gauge wires are thicker than the needles used for cytology, local anaesthesia with 1–2 ml of 2% lignocaine hydrochloride is preferable. In most women there is little or no sensation in the breast tissue itself so local anaesthesia may be limited to the skin. Because the puncture site does not overlie the lesion (due to the inserting angle of the needle), the local anaesthesia does not interfere with the image quality (Fig. 2.13).

If the biopsy is to be performed soon after localisation, dyes such as indigo-carmine[16], toluidine blue[17], methylene blue[18] or isosulfan[19] can be used instead of a wire. For this method, it is necessary also to mark the position of the lesion on the skin to guide the surgeon. As soon as the dye injection is begun the lesion is obscured because of a small amount of air in the needle, but a further 0.3–0.5 ml of dye must be injected to stain the area adequately.

Other interventional methods

A Tru-cut biopsy can be performed if histological examination is needed and excision is inappropriate. An automatic biopsy gun (Biopty® Bard) simplifies the procedure. Local anaesthesia is necessary and a small skin incision makes the needle insertion easier.

Ultrasound has also been reported as useful for localising breast tissue expander valves[20].

Fig. 2.13
Localisation
This echo poor mass lying deep in the breast was not palpable. Malignancy was suspected because of its lobulated shape and the posterior shadowing. Preoperative localisation was performed using a curved-end wire. The tip of the needle is advanced into the lesion, as shown; next the outer cannula is withdrawn and the wire is left in situ. Histology on the excised specimen revealed a complex lesion, consisting of a fibroadenoma together with a lobular carcinoma.

SCF: subcutaneous fat
GI: mammary gland

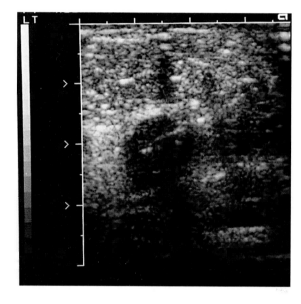

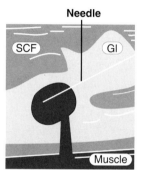

REFERENCES

1. B.D. Fornage, O. Toubas, M. Morel: Clinical, mammographic, and sonographic determination of preoperative breast cancer size. Cancer 60; 765–771, 1987.
2. J.W. Charboneau, C.C. Reading, T.J. Welch: CT and sonographically guided needle biopsy: current techniques and new innovations. AJR 154; 1–10, 1990.
3. D.B. Kopans, J.E. Meyer, K.K. Lindfors, S.S. Bucchianeri: Breast sonography to guide cyst aspiration and wire localisation of occult solid lesions. AJR 143; 489–492, 1984.
4. G. Rizzatto, L. Solbiati, F. Croce, E. Derchi: Aspiration biopsy of superficial lesions: ultrasonic guidance with a linear-array probe. AJR 148; 623–625, 1987.
5. B.D. Fornage, M.J. Faroux, A. Simatos: Breast masses: US-guided fine-needle aspiration biopsy. Radiology 162; 409–414, 1987.
6. B.D. Fornage, N. Sneige, M.J. Faroux, E. Andry: Sonographic appearance and ultrasound-guided fine-needle aspiration biopsy of breast carcinomas smaller than 1 cm^3. J Ultrasound Med 9; 559–568, 1990.
7. C. Hermamsen, H. Skovgaard, J. Jensen, et al: Diagnostic reliability of combined physical examination, mammography, and fine-needle puncture ('triple-test') in breast tumours — a prospective study. Cancer 60; 1866–1871,1987.
8. K. Dowlatshahi, H.J. Gent, R. Schmidt, et al: Nonpalpable breast tumors: diagnosis with stereotaxic localisation and fine-needle aspiration. Radiology 170; 427–433, 1989.
9. W.P. Evans, S.H. Cade: Needle localisation and fine-needle aspiration biopsy of nonpalpable breast lesions with use of standard and stereotactic equipment. Radiology 173; 53–56, 1989.
10. E.H. Smith: The hazard of fine-needle aspiration biopsy.

Ultrasound Med Biol 10; 629–634, 1984.
11. C. Nolsøe, L. Nielsen, S. Torp-Pederson, H.H. Holm: Major complications and deaths due to interventional ultrasonography: a review of 8000 cases. J Clin Ultrasound 18; 179–184, 1990.
12. D.B. Kopans, W.J. Gallagher, C.A. Swann, et al: Does preoperative needle localisation lead to an increase in local breast cancer recurrence? Radiology 167; 667–668, 1988.
13. D.B. Kopans, J.E. Meyer: Versatile spring hookwire breast lesion localizer. AJR 138; 586–587, 1982.
14. M.J. Homer, E.R. Pile-Spellman: Needle localisation of occult breast lesions with a curved-end retractable wire: technique and pitfalls. Radiology 161; 547–548, 1986.
15. E.J. Urrutia, M.C. Hawkins, B.G. Steinbach, et al: Retractable-barb needle for breast lesion localisation: use in 60 cases. Radiology 169; 845–847, 1988.
16. E. Ueno, Y. Aiyoshi, A. Imamura, et al: Ultrasonically guided biopsy of nonpalpable lesions of the breast by the spot method. Surg Gynecol Obstet 170; 153–155, 1990.
17. D.J. Czarnecki, H.K. Feider, G.F. Splittgerber: Toluidine blue dye as a breast localisation marker. AJR 153; 261–263, 1989.
18. J.I. Hirsch, W.L. Banks, J.S. Sullivan, J.S. Horsley: Effect of methylene blue on estrogen-receptor activity. Radiology 171; 105–107, 1989.
19. J.I. Hirsch, W.L. Banks, J.S. Sullivan, J.S. Horsley: Noninterference of isosulfan blue on estrogen-receptor activity. Radiology 171; 109–110, 1989.
20. E.K. Darnell, R.V. Demars: Ultrasonographic localization of breast tissue expander valves. J Ultrasound Med 6; 531–534, 1987.

Chapter 3

Anatomy and normal appearances

3.1 EMBRYOLOGY

During the fourth week of the embryonal life, enlargement of the single layered ectoderm forms the mammary streak (Fig. 3.1) and cell proliferation forms a slightly elevated area along a line extending from the axilla to the inguinal region; it is known as the milk line (see Fig. 3.21)[1, 2]. Unequal proliferation occurs at intervals along the line but, in humans, the intermediate portion of the cephalic one-third of the milk line eventually thickens to become the mammary primordium. Occasionally more than one pair of thickenings persists to form one or more rudimentary breasts (supernumerary breast; see Ch. 3.6). The mammary anlage increases its thickness and eventually epithelial buds sprout. They penetrate the mammary fat pad precursor tissues, branch and form about 20 epithelial cords. During the third trimester these solid cords become canalised by intercellular vacuolation and fusion of these vacuoles. Further epithelial differentiation occurs under hormonal stimulation (oestrogen, progesterone, prolactin, insulin and aldosterone) to form end-vesicles that contain colostrum. This colostral milk may be secreted for a few days after birth, stimulated by withdrawal of the maternal and placental hormones and secretion of fetal prolactin ('witch's milk'). Temporary hypertrophy of breasts of the fetus has been reported on ultrasound scans during the second trimester[3].

At the same time as the epithelium develops, mesenchymal differentiation also occurs to form several layers of fibroblasts attached to the epithelium. The mammary fat pad precursor tissue forms posterior to the epithelium; this is thought to trigger epithelial development. Mesenchymal cell proliferation around the mammary cord causes elevation of the epidermis and forms the nipple.

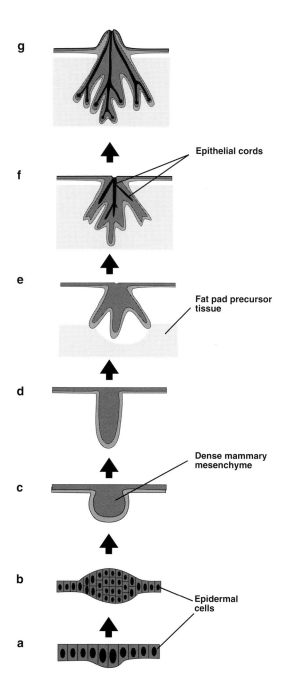

Fig. 3.1
Development of the mammary gland
a. mammary streak.
b. mammary ridge stage.
c. globular stage.
d. bud stage.
e. branching stage.
f. canalisation stage.
g. end vesicle stage.

REFERENCES

1. J. Russo, I.H. Russo: Development of the human mammary gland. In: The Mammary Gland, edited by M.C. Neville and C.W. Daniel. Plenum Press, New York, 1987, pp 67–93.
2. T. Sakakura: Mammary embryogenesis. In: The Mammary Gland, edited by M.C. Neville and C.W. Daniel. Plenum Press, New York, 1987, pp 37–66.
3. M. Bezzi, D.G. Mitchell, A.B. Kurtz, et al: Prominent fetal breasts — a normal variant. J Ultrasound Med 6; 655–658, 1987.

3.2 TOPOGRAPHIC ANATOMY

The breast lies on the chest wall extending from the level of the second or third rib to that of the sixth or seventh costal cartilage, from the sternal edge medially to the midaxillary line laterally; it lies mostly over the pectoralis major muscle (Fig. 3.2)[4]. This muscle arises from the clavicle, and from the sternal and costal cartilages; as it passes laterally, it thickens under the upper-outer quadrant of the breast and attaches to the anterolateral part of the upper humerus. The pectoralis minor muscle, lying deep to pectoralis major, arises from the medial end of the third to fifth ribs and attaches to the coracoid process of the scapula. Although small and of variable size, pec-

toralis minor is an important landmark for subdividing the levels of the axillary lymph nodes that are important in the staging of breast carcinoma (see Ch. 3.4). Part of the lower-outer quadrant of the breast lies on the serratus anterior muscle. All these muscles separate the gland from the rib cage itself.

The mammary gland is entirely contained within the layers of the superficial fascia and lies over the deep pectoral fascia (muscular fascia). The gland is usually thicker in its upper-outer quadrant, from where there is an extension towards the axilla (the axillary tail of Spence).

Fig. 3.2
Relationship between the breast and the chest wall muscles
The breast lies mainly over pectoralis major muscle with serratus anterior forming part of its bed inferolaterally. The pectoralis minor muscle lies deep to the pectoralis major muscle.

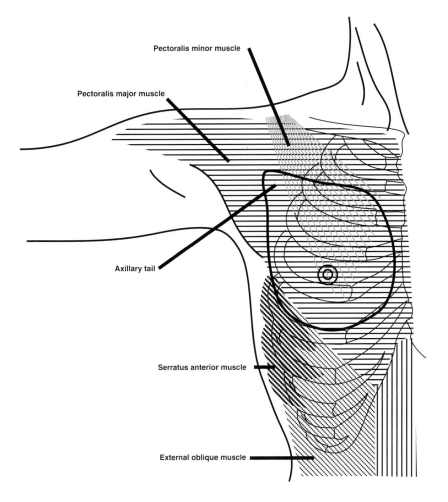

REFERENCES

4. C.D. Schneck, D.A. Lehman: Sonographic anatomy of the breast. Seminars in Ultrasound 3; 13–33, 1982.

3.3 SECTIONAL ANATOMY

The most superficial layer is the skin, composed of dermis and epidermis (Figs 3.3 and 3.4). The skin itself is difficult to visualise with direct contact scans (Fig. 3.5.a), but it can be observed as an echogenic layer when scanning through a stand-off (Fig. 3.5.b). The skin is slightly thicker in young women than in the elderly but is normally less than 3 mm, though the areolar skin is thicker. A relatively echo-poor line may be demonstrated within the skin layer, lying between the bright skin/stand-off echo and the dermis/subcutaneous fat interface echoes. An early report claimed that this double line indicated pathological thickening[5], but with modern high resolution transducers it can be observed in the normal breast.

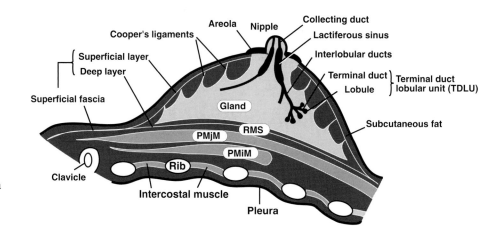

Fig. 3.3
Sectional anatomy of the breast (sagittal section)
The gland is encapsulated by the superficial and deep layers of the superficial fascia. Cooper's ligaments (suspensory ligaments of the gland) attach to the superficial layer of the superficial fascia. The fat layer between the posterior surface of the gland and the muscular fascia is known as the retromammary space; the deep layer of the superficial fascia lies within it.

Some 20 ducts open onto the nipple; they widen in the subareolar regions to form the lactiferous sinuses. Distally the ducts arborise into numerous interlobular ducts which lead into the terminal duct lobular units, the secretory portions.

RMS: retromammary space
PMiM: pectoralis minor muscle
PMjM: pectoralis major muscle

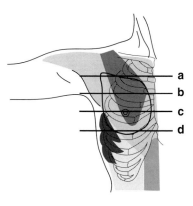

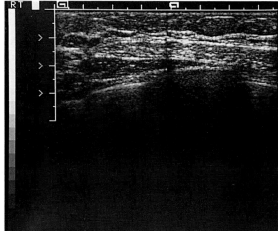

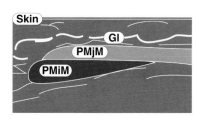

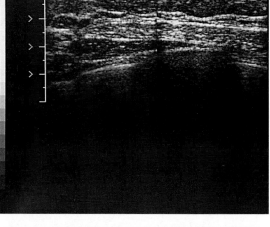

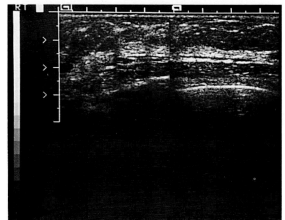

Fig. 3.4
Normal breast
a. In the upper part of the breast, the glandular tissue is thin while the pectoralis muscles are thicker. The reflectivity of the muscles is quite variable, tending to be echo-poor in young women but more reflective in older or obese women.
b. The mammary gland is seen as an echogenic layer. The two layers of the superficial fascia may be visualised, the superficial layer in the subcutaneous fat and the deep layer in the retromammary space. The suspensory ligaments (of Cooper) extend from the surface of the gland and attach to the superficial layer.

c. The nipple often causes shadowing because of its protruding shape and its fibrous or muscular components.
d. In the inferior part of the breast, serratus anterior muscle is seen laterally.

DL: deep layer of the superficial fascia
Gl: mammary gland
PMiM: pectoralis minor muscle
PMjM: pectoralis major muscle
RMS: retromammary space
SAM: serratus anterior muscle
SCF: subcutaneous fat
SL: superficial layer of the superficial fascia

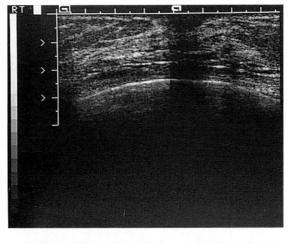

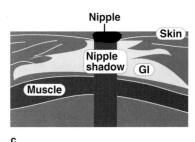

c

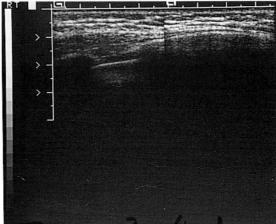

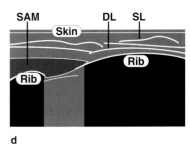

d

Fig. 3.5
The layers of the skin
The skin itself is difficult to visualise with the transducer in direct contact with the skin (**a**) but, when a stand-off is used, it is clearly seen as an echogenic band between the two bright echoes that represent the stand-off/epidermis and dermis/fat interfaces (**b**).

LD: lactiferous duct
SCF: subcutaneous fat

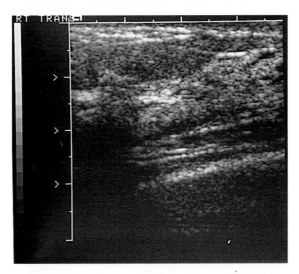

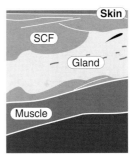

a

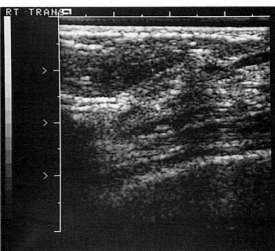

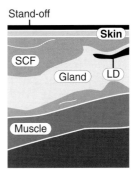

b

The mammary gland itself is enclosed by the two layers of the superficial fascia: the superficial and deep layers. While these are not always visualised, they can often be observed as fine echogenic lines when the ultrasound beam is orientated to be at right angles to the fascia (Fig. 3.6). Between the skin and the surface of the mammary gland lies the echo-poor subcutaneous fatty tissue.

The gland is composed of two histological types of tissue: the epithelial elements, comprising ducts and acini, and the stroma. The former consists of 15–20 branching glandular trees, each with a separate opening onto the nipple. The distal portions end in structures known as 'terminal duct lobular units' (TDLUs) (Fig. 3.3) which are the secreting units of the breast that produce milk during pregnancy and lactation. Both the TDLUs and the interlobular ducts are lined by a double layer of cells comprising an inner epithelial layer and an outer layer of myoepithelial cells (Plate P.3.1) which are histologically identical in the two locations in the resting state, despite the fundamental physiological differences between them. The interlobular mammary stroma consists of fibrous and adipose tissue of nondescript appearance. The intralobular stroma, however, has a different character, being composed of loosely textured fibrous tissue that contains lymphocytes, histiocytes, plasma cells and mast cells (Plate P.3.2). On ultrasound, the epithelial and connective tissue elements usually cannot be differentiated from each other and the whole of the glandular portion is strongly echogenic (Fig. 3.7). However, the normal glandular tissue may show much variation, as discussed later (see Ch. 3.5).

Between the posterior surface of the gland and the muscular fascia overlying the pectoralis major muscle (deep fascia), there is a layer of fatty tissue called the retromammary space.

The nipple itself and the tissue just deep to it are usually difficult to assess on ultrasound because of the so-called 'nipple shadow' (Fig. 3.8.a). One cause of this shadowing is nipple protrusion which not only interferes with proper contact between the skin and the transducer but also produces edge shadows (Fig. 3.8.b). In addition, the abundant connective tissues and muscle fibres within the nipple also cause attenuation. When examined carefully, the nipple is seen as a homogeneous round or oval area with slightly or markedly lower reflectivity than the skin layer. In the subareolar region, the ducts are wider in calibre; they are known as the lactiferous sinuses and are often seen as multiple anechoic tubular structures of up to a few millimetres in diameter behind the areola, converging on the nipple (Fig. 3.8.c).

Fig. 3.6
The two layers of the superficial fascia

The two layers of the superficial fascia are seen as bright lines in the subcutaneous and retromammary fatty tissue (**a**). The deep layer is better observed in the involuted breast when the retromammary space is more prominent (**b**).
In (**b**), the pectoralis muscle is highly reflective (echogenic). This is often seen in older and obese women.

DL: deep layer of the superficial fascia
Gl: mammary gland
RMS: retromammary space
SCF: subcutaneous fat
SL: superficial layer of the superficial fascia.

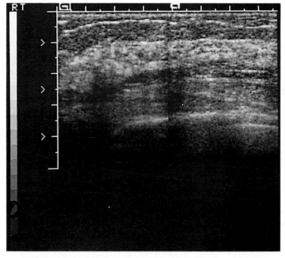
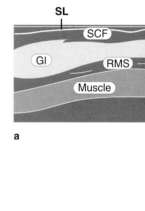

a

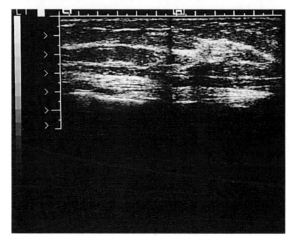
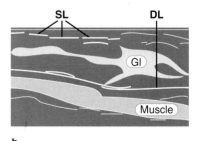

b

Fig. 3.7
The normal mammary gland
The mammary gland is more echogenic than the fat in the subcutaneous or retromammary spaces.

DL: deep layer of the superficial fascia
SL: superficial layer of the superficial fascia

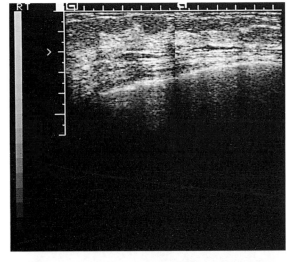

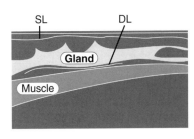

Fig. 3.8
The nipple
a. The nipple may cause shadowing and interfere with imaging of the tissues immediately deep to it. The skin of the areola is slightly thicker than that of the surrounding area.
b. Carefully examined, the nipple is seen as a homogeneous, slightly echo-poor area compared with the glandular tissues. Note the edge shadows from both sides of the nipple. (Magnified scan.)
c. Lactiferous sinuses are observed in the subareolar region. The shadowing in this image occurred because the transducer was only contacted lightly with breast to avoid compressing the lactiferous sinuses.

ES: edge shadows
GI: mammary gland
LS: lactiferous sinus
SCF: subcutaneous fat

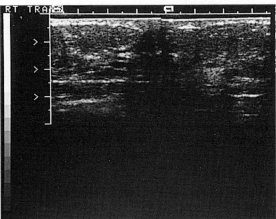

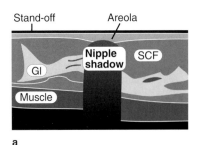

a

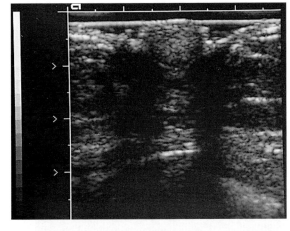

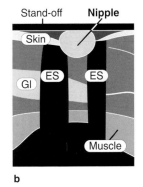

b

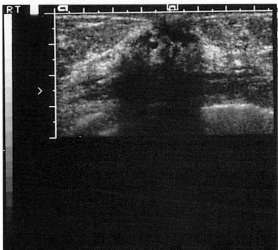

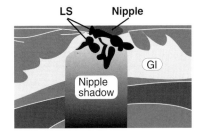

c

Cooper's ligaments are supportive structures that extend between the two layers of the superficial fascia. They are especially well seen on ultrasound in the partially involuted breast (Fig. 3.9.a). Although they appear as curvilinear echogenic lines between the glandular surface and the superficial layer of the superficial fascia, in fact they are thin membranes, curved in three dimensions. They commonly cause interface ('edge') shadows which may even occur when the ligaments themselves are not visualised (because they are aligned along the ultrasound beam) (Fig. 3.9.b). This type of shadowing is of no diagnostic significance and must be distinguished from shadows due to intraglandular lesions, as is typical of carcinomas. The fact that the shadowing originates anterior to the breast plate together with the scalloping of the fat/glandular tissue interface on either side of the shadows are helpful points of distinction[6].

Fig. 3.9
Cooper's ligaments
a. Cooper's ligaments are seen as curvilinear lines extending from the gland to the superficial layer of the superficial fascia.
b. Cooper's ligaments may cause fine linear shadows because of their alignment parallel to the ultrasound beam (interface or refractive shadows).

FI: fat island
GI: mammary gland
SCF: subcutaneous fat

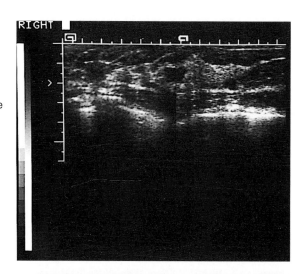
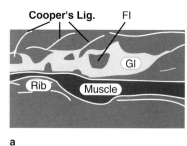

a

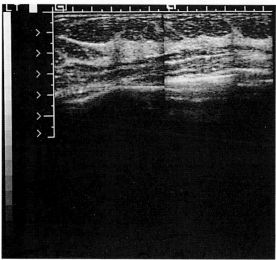
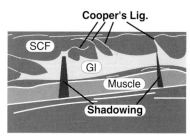

b

REFERENCES

5. D.B. Kopans, J.E. Meyer, K.H. Proppe: The double line of skin thickening of sonograms of the breast. Radiology 141: 485–487, 1981.
6. G. Kossoff: Causes of shadowing in breast sonography. Ultrasound Med Biol 14 (suppl 1); 211–215, 1988.

3.4 BLOOD SUPPLY

ARTERIES

The main arteries supplying the breast are branches of the lateral thoracic artery (also termed the external mammary artery) and perforating branches of the internal mammary artery (also termed the internal thoracic artery) (Fig. 3.10). The lateral thoracic artery arises from the axillary artery distal to the thoracoacromial artery; it passes inferiorly along the lateral border of the pectoralis major muscle and gives off lateral mammary branches, which turn around the lateral border of the pectoralis major muscle to supply the breast. The internal mammary artery arises from the first part of the subclavian artery and descends behind the cartilages of the upper ribs, where it lies slightly lateral to the sternum. Branches arise in the first to fourth intercostal spaces and penetrate the pectoralis major muscle to reach the deep surface of the gland along its medial edge. A small supply also comes from the pectoral branch of the thoracoacromial artery and from the intercostal arteries.

These vessels are regularly detected on colour Doppler studies (Plate C.5) and are occasionally imaged on real-time images as anechoic tubular structures. Colour Doppler displays vessels too small to be resolved on real-time; typically they lie within the glandular tissues, or run on the surface of the gland and in the Cooper's ligaments or fibrous tissue bands (Plate C.6.a). They undergo physiological dilatation just before or around the onset of menstruation[7], and particularly during pregnancy (Plate C.6.b) and lactation. Although there are considerable normal variations, the arterial patterns are usually symmetrical on the two sides[8].

VEINS

The venous drainage of the breast is important not only because veins are the route of haematogenous metastases from carcinomas but also because the lymphatic vessels generally follow the same course. The veins are divided into two systems: superficial and deep[9]. The superficial veins lie just deep to the superficial fascia and are occasionally observed on ultrasound when blood flow is increased, such as may occur in advanced carcinomas or inflammatory diseases (Fig. 4.19, Plate C.7.f). Subcutaneous lymphatic channels may also be dilated in these cases — a Doppler study may allow a distinction since lymphatics do not give Doppler signals. The superficial veins on the two sides communicate with each other.

The deep veins usually run alongside the arteries but are more variable in position. They drain into the internal mammary, axillary, subclavian veins and the azygous system via the intercostal veins. The intercostal veins anastomose with the vertebral veins and this route is considered to be responsible for bone metastases that bypass the pulmonary bed[10]. The superficial and deep veins anastomose with each other through the mammary gland.

Fig. 3.10
Arterial supply of the breast
The two dominant supplies come from the lateral thoracic and the internal mammary arteries. The thoracoacromial artery and intercostal arteries also provide small branches to the breast.

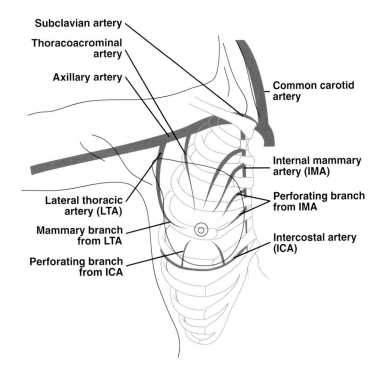

LYMPHATICS

In the breast subdermal and intramammary lymphatics anastomose at the subareolar plexus; flow is centrifugal, towards the axillary, internal mammary and intercostal chains[11] (Fig. 3.11).

The axillary chain forms the main drainage; the associated nodes are subdivided into the following groups:

- External mammary: lymph nodes along the lateral thoracic vein
- Scapular: lymph nodes along the subscapular vein
- Axillary: lymph nodes along the lateral portion of the axillary artery

- Central: lymph nodes embedded in fat in the centre of the axilla
- Subclavicular (or infraclavicular): lymph nodes along the subclavicular vein medial to the origin of the thoracoacromial artery
- Interpectoral nodes (Rotter): lymph nodes between the major and minor pectoral muscles along the pectoral branch of the thoracoacromial artery

For surgical purposes, the axillary lymph nodes are divided into three levels according to their relationship with the pectoralis minor muscle (Fig. 3.12). Nodes lying lateral to this muscle are termed level I, those deep to pectoralis minor are level II and those lying medial to it are level III. Level I and II lymph nodes are removed in

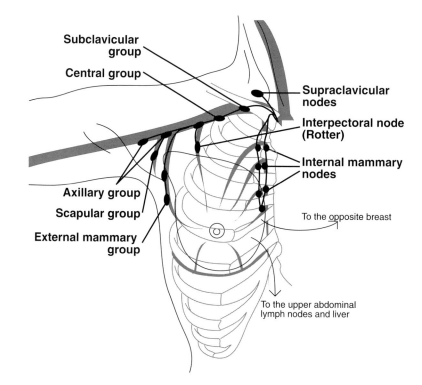

Fig. 3.11
Lymph nodes of the breast
External mammary: lymph nodes along the lateral thoracic vessels.
Scapular: lymph nodes along the subscapular vessels.
Axillary: lymph nodes along the lateral part of the axillary vessels.
Central: lymph nodes along the medial part of the axillary vessels.
Subclavicular: lymph nodes along the subclavian vessels.
Interpectoral (Rotter): lymph node between the pectoralis major and minor muscles.
Internal mammary: lymph nodes along the internal mammary vessels.
Supraclavicular: lymph nodes in the supraclavicular fossa.

Subclavicular group
Central group
Supraclavicular nodes
Interpectoral node (Rotter)
Internal mammary nodes
Axillary group
Scapular group
External mammary group
To the opposite breast
To the upper abdominal lymph nodes and liver

an extended total mastectomy (mastectomy with axillary dissection). Removal of the level III lymph nodes requires excision or division of the pectoralis minor muscle, as in radical mastectomy or Patey's modified radical mastectomy in which the pectoralis major muscle is preserved.

Involvement of the supraclavicular lymph nodes, unlike involvement of lymph nodes of the axillary chain, is considered as a distant metastasis because it occurs in a retrograde fashion from the lymph nodes at the jugulo-subclavian venous confluence.

The internal mammary lymph nodes accompany the internal mammary vessels and lie in the fat and areolar tissue behind the intercostal muscles in the intercostal spaces. In the upper three intercostal spaces these lymph nodes are situated immediately anterior to the parietal pleura but, below the fourth intercostal space, the transverse thoracic muscle intervenes between the internal mammary vessels and the parietal pleura. Lymph nodes may be found either medial or lateral to these vessels, but usually lie within 3 cm of the sternal edge[9]. Normal internal mammary nodes are not seen on ultrasound; lymph nodes containing metastases are usually impalpable, but can be imaged by parasternal ultrasound scans[12].

Intercostal lymph nodes lie posteriorly in the paravertebral region.

A small amount of the lymphatic flow from the breast crosses to the opposite side and some passes to the upper abdominal lymph nodes via diaphragmatic lymphatics.

Fig. 3.12
Subdivision of the axillary lymph nodes by levels
Level I: nodes lateral to pectoralis minor muscle.
Level II: nodes deep to pectoralis minor muscle.
Level III: nodes medial to pectoralis minor muscle.

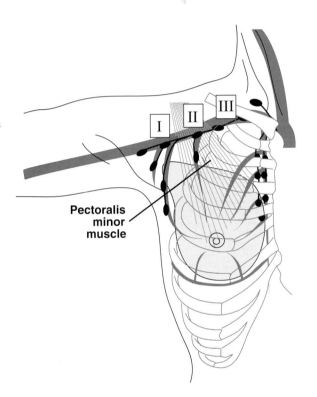

Pectoralis minor muscle

REFERENCES

7. M. Sambrook, J.C. Bamber, H. Minasian, C.R. Hill: Ultrasonic Doppler study of the hormonal response of blood flow in the normal human breast. Ultrasound Med Biol 13; 121–129, 1987.

8. P.N. Burns, J.D. Davies, M. Halliwell, et al: Doppler ultrasound in the diagnosis of breast cancer. In: Ultrasound in Breast and Endocrine Disease. Churchill Livingstone, New York, 1984, pp 41–56.

9. C.D. Haagensen: Diseases of the Breast (3rd edn). W.B. Saunders, Philadelphia, 1986, pp 20–24.

10. C.Q. Henriques: The veins of the vertebral column and their role in the spread of cancer. Ann R Coll Surg 31; 1–22, 1962.

11. J.S. Spratt: Anatomy of the breast. Major Prob Clin Surg 5; 1–13, 1979.

12. J.C. Scatarige, U.M. Hamper, S. Sheth, H.A. Allen III: Parasternal sonography of the internal mammary vessels: technique, normal anatomy, and lymphadenopathy. Radiology 172; 453–457, 1989.

3.5 NORMAL VARIATIONS AND AGE CHANGES

There is some difficulty in defining the limits of normality for the breast because so-called 'benign breast change' (see Ch. 6.2) is very common and is considered by some to be normal. The problem is evident both on histology and X-ray mammography. Similarly the 'normal' ultrasonic appearances also have a wide range of variation.

MATURE BREAST

To help understand the chronological changes in the breast, the ultrasonic appearances in the mature women of child-bearing age are described first. The glandular tissue is a fairly homogeneous, echogenic layer that is cone-shaped in the centre of the breast and sheet-like elsewhere (Fig. 3.13). It is typically thicker in the upper-outer quadrants. The gland is traversed by ducts that are sometimes observed as echo-free tubular structures 1–2 mm in diameter, more prominent centrally, while the wider lactiferous sinuses are usually apparent in the subareolar region. Anterior and posterior to the glandular cone are the echo-poor layers of fat in the subcutaneous and retromammary spaces. The subcutaneous space is traversed by the fine reflective lines of Cooper's ligaments

which often elevate the portion of the gland to which they are attached so that the anterior surface of the gland has a scalloped contour. Because of the way the breast is flattened against the chest wall when the patient is examined supine, the Cooper's ligaments tend to curve so that their superficial portions lie horizontally.

The reflectivity of the glandular tissue may be attributed to the numerous interfaces between the small constituent elements (ducts, connective tissue and acini); changes in the size, number, proportion or distribution of these elements alter their echo levels and their uniformity. When these changes are marked they may be classified as 'benign breast change'.

In one of the more common variations, small (1–2 mm) poorly reflective bands are scattered throughout the gland, especially in the relatively thicker portions of the upper-outer quadrants. These echo-poor areas tend to radiate from the nipple; they are probably attributable to periductal changes, such as fibrosis, or to adenosis (Fig. 3.14).

Another common variation is duct dilatation. Dilated ducts extend more widely than normal and are usually multiple, often also associated with nipple discharge. The

Fig. 3.13
Homogeneous glandular tissues
In breasts with homogeneously echogenic glands, such as in this subject, detecting an intraglandular lesion is relatively straightforward.

DL: deep layer of the superficial fascia
SL: superficial layer of the superficial fascia

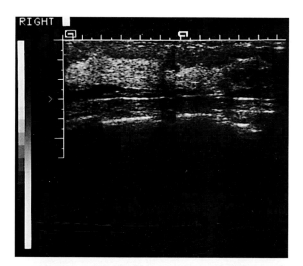
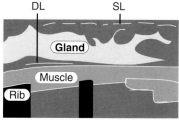

Fig. 3.14
Small echo-poor areas in the glandular tissue
Small echo-poor foci are often seen in the gland, giving it a mottled or spongy texture when they are scanned tangentially (★); scanned radially, they are seen as linear streaks (★★). These structures are probably due to periductal fibrotic stroma or adenosis.

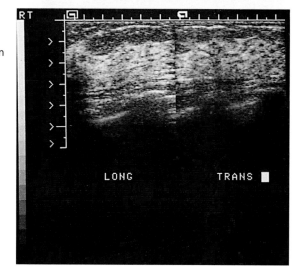
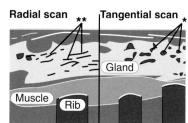

finding of a single dilated duct in a woman with nipple discharge suggests pathological changes such as an intraductal papilloma or carcinoma (see Ch. 5.3).

The reflectivity of the glandular tissue is also variable. While it is usually considerably more echogenic than the fatty tissue, this difference may be slight and occasionally the glandular tissue is isoechoic with the fatty tissue. This variety, the 'echo-poor gland', is more common in young women in whom the typical convex shape of the interface between the surface of the gland and the subcutaneous fat allows a distinction between the two components even though the reflectivity is similar.

PUBERTAL BREAST

In prepubertal children mammary gland development does little more than keep pace with the general growth of the body and the breast contains a few small ducts scattered throughout a fibrous stroma without formed lobules. One or two years before menarche, the glandular tissues enlarge rapidly. Under the coordinated action of several hormones, especially oestrogen and progesterone, the ducts lengthen and branch; subsequently lobules bud out. Occasionally these developments occur asymmetrically and a hard, discoid lump is felt in one breast, a condition known as 'unilateral early ripening'. This glandular tissue is observed as an echo-poor 'mass' beneath the nipple on ultrasound (Fig. 3.15) and must not be mistaken for a tumour because excision will remove all the glandular tissue and prevent development of the breast.

Fig. 3.15
Unilateral early ripening
This 8-year-old girl presented with a left breast lump. The normal glandular tissue is seen as an echo-poor 'mass' beneath the nipple.

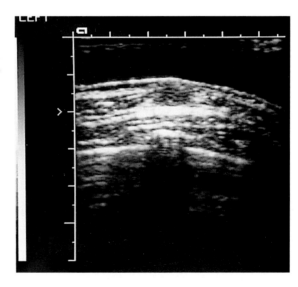
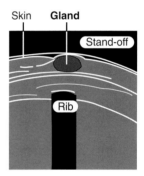

YOUNG WOMEN

In young women the glandular tissues are relatively thick and the subcutaneous and retromammary fat spaces are small (Fig. 3.16.a). The glandular tissue is usually of low reflectivity. In some subjects the glandular tissue is heterogeneous on ultrasound and occasionally this may form confusing echo-poor regions (Fig. 3.16.b); this is probably due to an imbalance in development of the different elements. In a common form the glandular tissue contains numerous scattered small echo-poor areas giving a mottled or spongiform pattern; this finding was previously described as a normal variation. In obese young women, the breasts may be largely occupied by fat, as in the involuted breast.

Fig. 3.16
A young woman's breast
a. Thick glandular tissue. The breast of this 21-year-old woman is almost completely occupied by glandular tissue; neither subcutaneous nor retromammary fatty layers are seen.
b. Echo-poor glandular tissues. The central glandular tissue of this 17-year-old woman is mainly echo-poor with more normal reflectivity at the periphery. Underdevelopment of the lobules in young women is considered to be the cause of this confusing appearance. A fibroadenoma is also seen on this scan.

Gl: mammary gland
Fa: fibroadenoma

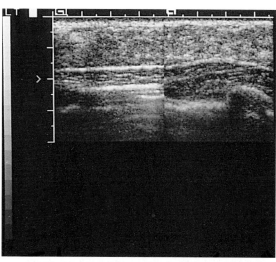
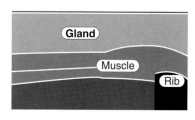

a

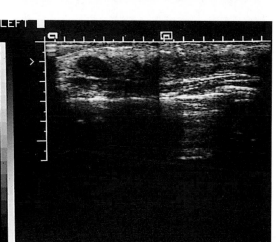
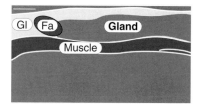

b

PREGNANCY AND LACTATION

During pregnancy there is considerable increase in the size of the terminal duct lobular units at the expense of the breast stroma and the epithelial elements come to occupy almost the entire breast which has very little fat (Plate P.3.3, Fig. 3.17). During lactation, the glandular tissue become poorly reflective and homogeneous with a fine texture, the 'ground glass' pattern (Fig. 3.18). The ducts are dilated.

Fig. 3.17
Pregnant breast
In pregnancy the glandular tissues increase in thickness. The texture of the gland becomes homogeneous.

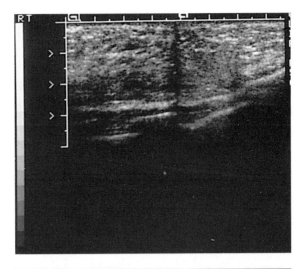
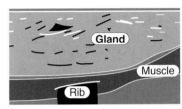

Fig. 3.18
Lactating breast
During lactation the glandular tissues are echo-poor with a fine, ground-glass pattern (**a**). Ducts become prominent (**b**).

SL: superficial layer of the superficial fascia
SCF: subcutaneous fat

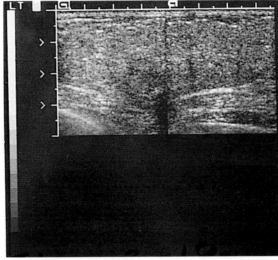
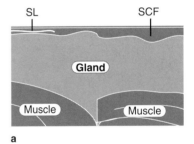

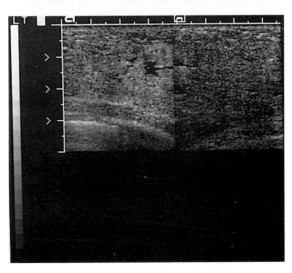
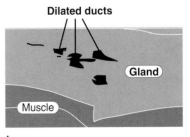

INVOLUTION

The age of onset and extent of involution vary markedly and are accelerated by ovarian ablation (by surgery, radiotherapy or chemotherapy) and inhibited by hormone replacement therapy. The thickness of the glandular tissue decreases and they form bright band-like structures within the fat, the two components being intermingled (Fig. 3.19). In extreme involution, the parenchymal elements are almost absent and only connective tissue strands remain as networks of intense linear echoes in the echo-poor fat. Mammography is particularly sensitive in the detection of very small lesions in such non-dense breasts, while the accuracy of ultrasound is neither improved nor reduced.

MALE BREAST

In the male the breast remains rudimentary with small ducts and little supporting tissue, seen as echogenic lines. Terminal duct lobular units are lacking and the band-like or cone-shaped glandular layer is not seen (Fig. 3.20).

Fig. 3.19
Involuted breast
During involution, the persisting glandular tissue is seen as thin echogenic strands that form networks around multiple 'fat islands'. Detection of lesions with the same reflectivity as the fat may be difficult in such a breast, though such lesions are relatively rare and are usually benign.

DL: deep layer of the superficial fascia
SL: superficial layer of the superficial fascia
FI: fat island
SCF: subcutaneous fat

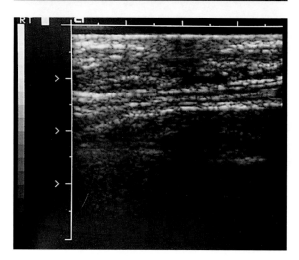

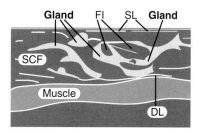

Fig. 3.20
Male breast
A cone or layer of the echogenic gland is lacking in the male breast. Only sparse fibrotic strands are seen.

SCF: subcutaneous fat

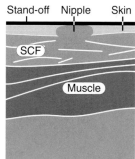

3.6 ANOMALIES

CLINICAL FEATURES

The commonest anomalies of the breast are listed in Table 3.1.

Amastia (complete absence of one or both breasts), absence of breast tissue or nipple, or rudimentary mammary gland are rare though sometimes are associated with underdevelopment or absence of structures of the shoulder girdle, chest or arm[13].

Accessory or supernumerary breasts (polymastia or pleomastia) are common (1–2%) and may involve any of the three components of the breast (the glandular parenchyma, the areola or the nipple) in any combination. They develop along the milk lines, which extend from the axilla to the groin (Fig. 3.21). The commonest is an accessory nipple (polythelia), which occurs in both sexes and is most common just below the normal breast. Accessory mammary glands are most often located in the axilla; they enlarge as the normal breast tissue develops and become especially prominent during pregnancy and lactation. If the ductal structures are complete they secrete milk but, when the accessory glandular tissue develops without a nipple or areola, it forms a mass which is often misinterpreted as a lipoma or other solid benign tumour. The same pathologies as affect the normal gland (e.g. carcinomas, benign tumours, benign mammary change) also occur in the accessory gland.

Some developmental anomalies are associated with endocrine abnormalities. Hypoplasia may be related to ovarian dysfunction, especially in Turner's syndrome. Hormonally active tumours produce enlargement of breast tissue by causing precocious puberty. Hypertrophy unassociated with an identified hormonal abnormality may occur in adolescents and often needs surgical reduction.

Congenital nipple flattening or inversion must be differentiated from acquired retraction of the nipple, which may be caused by a carcinoma or by duct ectasia.

Table 3.1 Breast anomalies
Formative anomalies
Absent, or rudimentary, breast—rare
Amastia (complete absence of breast)—very rare
Absence of the nipple
Absent, or rudimentary, mammary gland
Supernumerary breast
Accessory breast (1–2%)—affects gland, areola or nipple singly or in combination
Developmental anomalies
Hypoplasia
Idiopathic
Ovarian dysfunction, e.g. Turner's syndrome
Hyperplasia
Precocious puberty, idiopathic (constitutional) ovarian tumours or granulosa cell tumours
Gynaecomastia (see Ch. 6.3)
Early development (see Ch. 3.5.2)
Hypertrophy (adolescent)
Abnormal shape
Nipple flattening or inversion

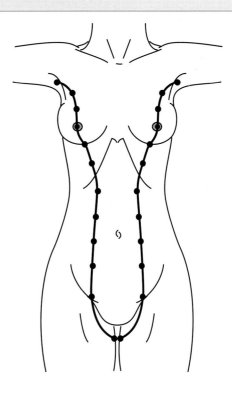

Fig. 3.21
Milk line
The milk line extends from the axilla to the inguinal region, the site of the mammary ridge in the embryo; accessory glands occur along this line.

ULTRASOUND FEATURES

Most changes are self-evident clinically so that investigations are not needed.

An accessory gland may present as a mass; it is seen as a region with the same echogenic structure as the normal gland (Fig. 3.22) and ultrasound is useful in distinguishing it from a lipoma or other tumour. An accessory gland can be differentiated from the axillary tail, a normal extension of the glandular tissue towards the axilla, because the accessory gland is separated from the main gland (see Ch. 3.2). An inverted nipple is seen as an echo-poor area, its flat shape being less attenuating than an everted nipple (Fig. 3.23).

Fig. 3.22
Accessory gland
This woman noticed a lump in the right axilla. On ultrasound, an echogenic area with the same appearances as the normal glandular tissue is seen lying lateral to the normal gland.

FI: fat island
GI: mammary gland
PMiM: pectoralis minor muscle
PMjM: pectoralis major muscle

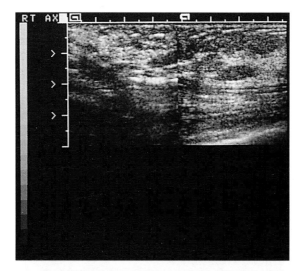

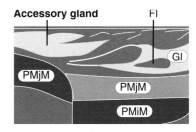

Fig. 3.23
Inverted nipple
An inverted nipple is seen as an echo-poor nodule on ultrasound. Because it is flat, shadowing is less intense than from a normal everted nipple.

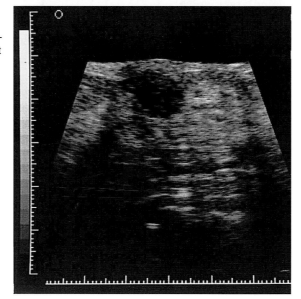

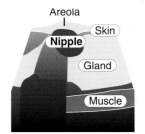

REFERENCES

13. C.D. Haagensen: Diseases of the Breast (3rd edn). W.B. Saunders, Philadelphia, 1986, pp 20–24.

Chapter 4

Diagnostic features on ultrasound

The pathological changes affecting the breast are complex and sometimes confusing. While most malignancies in the breast are primary tumours of various histological types, metastases being rare, benign changes are much more varied; they include benign tumours, infection, the effects of trauma, including surgery and 'benign breast change'. This wide variety of pathology means that the corresponding range of ultrasonic features is complex. The typical appearances of each condition are described later; in this chapter an approach to the interpretation of ultrasound images is offered, together with an evaluation of the significance of the individual diagnostic features.

From the ultrasonic point of view, breast diseases can be divided into two groups: those that produce a mass and disorders without a mass.

MASSES

Most breast diseases, especially neoplasms, form masses that can be visualised on ultrasound. The important diagnostic features are listed in Table 4.1. The morphological features are divided into primary (the features of masses themselves) and secondary (those produced by interaction with the surrounding tissues). Morphological abnormalities are the most important diagnostic features but additional information from dynamic tests and Doppler signals are useful, especially in atypical or equivocal cases.

Morphological features

Primary features

Shape
Masses can be described as round, oval, lobulated or irregular in shape. A rounded shape is typical of small or tense cysts (Fig. 4.1.a) and may also be seen in small carcinomas. Lax cysts and fibroadenomas are typical examples of oval lesions (Fig. 4.1.b). A lobulated shape is typical of clusters of cysts (Fig. 4.1.c) and of fibroadenomas; it is occasionally seen in circumscribed carcinomas, though an irregular shape is more typical (Fig. 4.1.d).

Table 4.1 Ultrasound features of mass lesions in the breast			
	Benign	**Indeterminate**	**Malignant**
Morphological features			
Primary features of the mass			
Shape	Round, oval	Lobulated	Irregular
D:W ratio	<0.8		>0.8
Internal echoes			
Intensity	None, high	Fatty tissue, low	Very low
Texture	Uniform	Heterogeneous	
Calcification echoes	None	Coarse bright echoes	Small bright
Cystic change or intracystic tumour	May be seen		May be seen
Intracystic echoes	Fat–fluid level		Fluid–fluid level
Lesion margin			
Regularity	Smooth		Irregular
Definition	Well-defined		Ill-defined
Edge shadows	(Present)		(Absent)
Halo	(Absent)		(Present)
Posterior echoes	Enhancement	No change	Shadowing
Secondary features in the surrounding tissues			
Adjacent structures	Stretched		Interrupted
Subcutaneous fat echoes intensity	No change		Increased
Duct dilatation	(Absent)		(Present)
Venous or lymphatic dilatation	(Absent)		(Present)
Skin thickening	(Absent)		(Present)
Lymphadenopathy	Undetectable		(Present)
Dynamic tests			
Compressibility	Compressible		Incompressible
Mobility	Mobile		Fixed
Fixation to the fascia	(Absent)		May be fixed
Doppler features			
Vascularity	No change	Slightly increased	Increased
Flow pattern	Normal		Disturbed
Flow velocity	Normal		High
PI (pulsatility index)	Normal		Low

(Absent) or (Present) indicates variable features.

Fig. 4.1
Variations in shape

a. Round cyst with inspissated material. This lesion is round and has smooth margins with edge shadows. The glandular layer is smoothly compressed at its anterior surface to form an echogenic rim. These appearances suggest a benign lesion but it is not echo-free and there is slight posterior attenuation. Because of these atypical feature this lesion was aspirated under ultrasound guidance; thick yellow paste was retrieved.

b. Oval fibroadenoma. The oval shape, smooth margin and homogeneous internal texture of this lesion are the typical features of a fibroadenoma.

c. Lobulated cyst. Lobulated cysts are in fact a cluster of oval cysts and are quite common.

d. Carcinoma of irregular shape. An irregularly shaped mass with an echogenic halo (boundary echoes) and posterior attenuation are the typical features of a carcinoma.

DL: deep layer of the superficial fascia
ES: edge shadow
Fa: fibroadenoma
Gl: mammary gland
PE: posterior enhancement
SCF: subcutaneous fat
SL: superficial layer of the superficial fascia

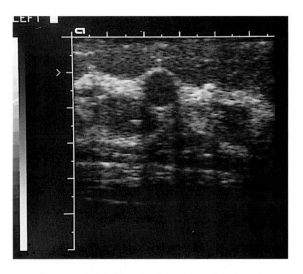
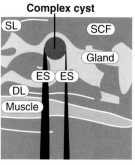

a

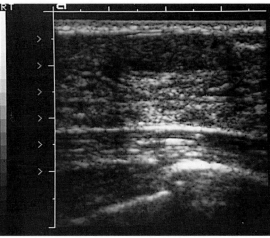
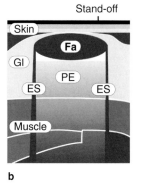

b

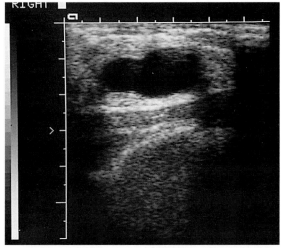
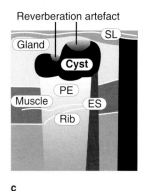

c

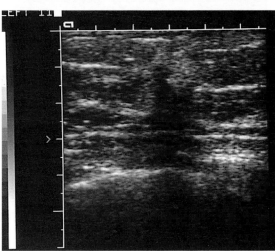
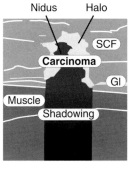

d

Masses tend to adopt a characteristic lie in the breast tissues with their long axis lying parallel or at right angles to the skin. This can be quantified by the ratio of the AP to the transverse diameters. This was first described by Tajima et al[1] as the longitudinal:transverse ratio, an unintuitive designation that has now been changed to the depth:width (D:W) ratio. Benign lesions, especially fibroadenomas and focal benign mammary change, are usually soft and thus are flattened by the pressure of the transducer; they tend to expand within the normal structures and, because they are mobile, they settle within the glandular tissue when the patient is supine (Fig. 4.2) so that their depth is almost always less than their width (D:W ratio <0.8) (Fig. 4.3.a). On the other hand, in malignancies, the D:W ratio may be 1.0 or even greater because of their incompressibility, invasive growth pattern and fixation to the surrounding structures (Fig. 4.3.b). The high D:W ratio is most obvious in small carcinomas (<2 cm), where it is a particularly useful diagnostic feature because many of the other signs of malignancy may not have developed. Larger carcinomas, however, tend to revert to the flat position with lower D:W ratios, so the sign becomes less useful.

Fig. 4.2
Depth:width ratio
Benign lesions usually have a small D:W ratio because they are soft and so are compressed by the transducer; in addition they grow within the normal architecture of the breast and they are mobile and so align with the fibrous layers of the breast, which are horizontal when the patient is supine.

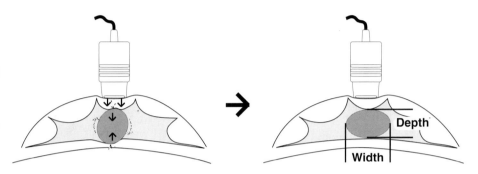

Fig. 4.3
The depth:width ratio

This cyst (**a**) measures 2.5 cm × 0.8 cm giving a D:W ratio of 0.3, a benign sign. It is surrounded by glandular tissue which remains intact. The D:W ratio of the small carcinoma in (**b**) is 0.8/0.6 = 1.3. This is above the upper limit for benign lesions (>0.8) and the appearance is very suspicious, despite its homogeneous internal texture and lack of posterior shadowing.

D: depth
SCF: subcutaneous fat
W: width

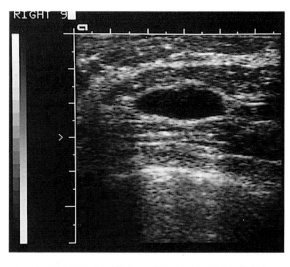

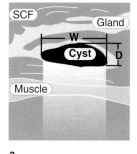

a

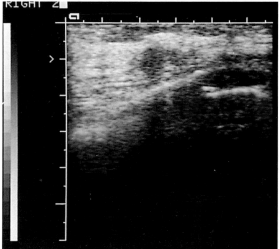

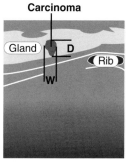

b

Internal echoes

The internal echoes of a lesion can be classified according to their intensity and homogeneity. Additional features include calcifications, cystic changes, intracystic masses and intracystic echoes.

The internal echogenicity is best evaluated by comparison with the echogenicity of the adjacent subcutaneous fat; anechoic, very echo-poor, echo-poor, isoechoic and echogenic masses can be distinguished. For practical purposes, absence of echoes ('anechoic' or 'echo-free') indicates clear fluid; the ultrasound diagnosis of anechoic cysts is straightforward (Fig. 4.4.a) although cysts are not always echo-free. Purely cellular tumours, such as lymphomas, have been reported to be 'anechoic' but this appearance is very rare and usually low level echoes can, in fact, be demonstrated within them.

Lesions with 'very low' internal echoes appear darker than the fatty tissues but are not anechoic, while 'low' is used to describe lesions that are slightly less echogenic than fatty tissue. The importance of this distinction lies in the fact that most malignancies have very low internal echoes (Fig. 4.4.b) while fibroadenomas usually show low

Fig. 4.4
Range of echoes of masses

a. Echo-free cyst. Complete absence of echoes is almost pathognomonic of a cyst. In this example, the diagnosis of a simple cyst is supported by the posterior enhancement and the thin, smooth wall.

b. Carcinoma with very low level echoes. Carcinomas often have very weak echoes because the fibrous tissue they contain absorbs the ultrasound beam strongly. The posterior attenuation and irregular shape are also typical features of a carcinoma.

c. Fibroadenoma with low level echoes. This lesion has definite internal echoes, though they are weaker than those of the surrounding fatty tissue. Low intensity echoes are typical of fibroadenomas.

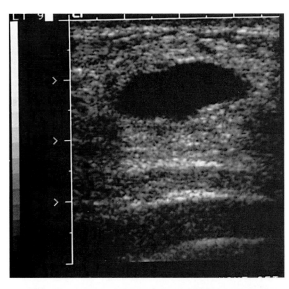

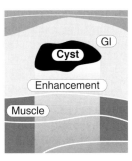

a

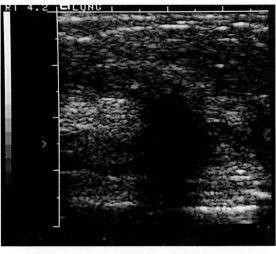

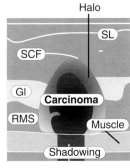

b

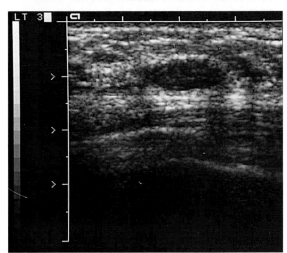

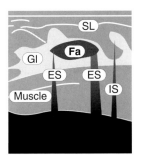

c

internal echoes (Fig. 4.4.c). 'Isoechoic' masses (where the reflectivity equals that of fat) include fibroadenomas (Fig. 4.4.d), lipomas and lymph nodes; carcinomas are rarely as echogenic as fat, an exception being colloid carcinoma. Lesions that are isoechoic with the surrounding tissue may be difficult to detect, especially in the involuted breast where fat has replaced the glandular tissue. Demonstration of the margin in its entirety is important to differentiate a true lesion from a fat island (see Ch. 2); here, too, examination during palpation and observation of the difference of consistency between a lesion and the surrounding tissue under dynamic compression are useful because fat is readily compressible.

Echogenic breast masses are rare; lipomas (Fig. 4.4.e) and granulomas are typical examples, while fibroadenomas and carcinomas with extensive microcalcification may occasionally return such strong echoes.

d. Fibroadenoma with the same echo intensity as fatty tissue.
Fibroadenomas of this type are easily missed on ultrasound, especially in involuted breasts, because they simulate a fat island. Their detection and differentiation depend on dynamic tests: fibroadenomas are freely mobile and relatively incompressible whereas fat is readily compressible but relatively immobile. In addition, fat does not produce the distal enhancement that is often found with fibroadenomas.

e. Lipoma with high level echoes.
Lipomas are often more echogenic than the surrounding fatty tissue, presumably because they also contain fibrous tissue. This lesion lies anterior to the superficial fascia where there is no glandular tissue, confirming the diagnosis.

ES: edge shadow
Fa: fibroadenoma
Gl: mammary gland
IS: interface shadows from Cooper's ligaments
RMS: retromammary space
SCF: subcutaneous fat
SL: superficial layer of the superficial fascia

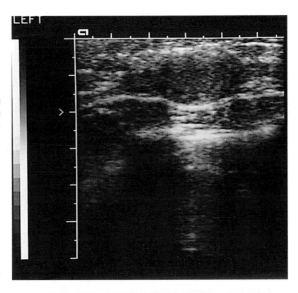

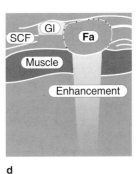

d

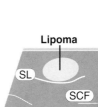

e

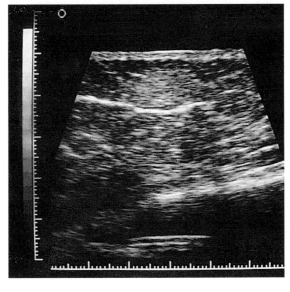

Fibroadenomas and complex cysts are usually homogeneous in texture (Fig. 4.5.a), whereas most malignancies have heterogeneous internal echoes (Fig. 4.5.b). Generally, the larger the tumour, the more heterogeneous the internal echoes, presumably because of varying proportions of cells and stroma and because of necrosis or haemorrhage in the lesion.

Calcification may occur in both benign and malignant lesions. The calcification associated with malignancy typically forms numerous small foci (<1 mm in diameter) that may lie within the tumour or in the surrounding breast. It is elegantly demonstrated on mammograms as 'microcalcification'. On ultrasound punctate echogenicities without distal shadowing are found. They are more readily detected when they are clumped together, as is frequently the case, and when they lie within a tumour mass, because their intense echoes stand out in contrast with the echo-poor background (Fig. 4.6.a)[2]. Microcalcifications lying in the glandular tissue are masked by the echogenicity of the normal gland and are therefore very difficult to detect. This problem largely accounts for the limitations of ultrasound in screening for breast

Fig. 4.5
Homogeneity of the internal echoes
a. Fibroadenoma with uniform internal echoes. This slightly lobulated lesion has very homogeneous internal echoes, a typical feature of a fibroadenoma.
b. Carcinomas, especially large ones, have heterogeneous internal echoes because of fibrosis, necrosis and calcification. In this case, a large necrotic region produces a cystic space, an unusual feature.

ES: edge shadow
Fa: fibroadenoma
SCF: subcutaneous fat

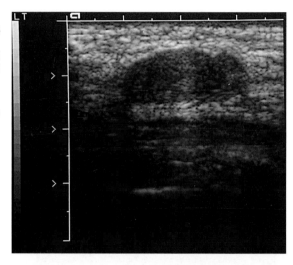
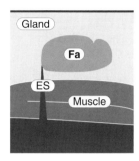

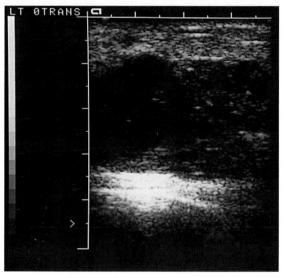
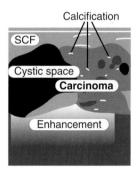

cancer. Calcification within the glandular tissue occurs around carcinomas (actually an extension of the tumour) and in benign breast change (Fig. 4.6.b).

The number and size of the bright echoes do not correlate well with the true number or size of calcifications detected on histological specimens or on mammograms; they usually seem fewer and larger on ultrasound because tiny single foci are missed and only larger or clumped calcifications are detected. The size of the bright spots on ultrasound scans is determined by the spatial resolution of the scanner (limited by the beam width) and by the intensity of the reflections, both of which tend to make them appear larger than they actually are. Although tumours themselves may cause attenuative shadows, shadowing from malignant calcification is not commonly observed because the foci are smaller than the width of the ultrasound beam.

Calcification in benign tumours is usually coarse and often produces shadowing (Fig. 4.6.c). Curvilinear calcification on the surface of the fibroadenomas is a typical example of the benign pattern.

Fig. 4.6
Calcification
Microcalcification within carcinomas is seen as small bright echoes that lack shadows (**a**), but when scattered in the glandular tissue it is very difficult to recognise (**b**) because both have high level echoes and the small calcifications do not cast acoustic shadows. Coarse calcification forms larger foci that cast shadows (**c**) (in a fibroadenoma in this case). Fibroadenomas tend to calcify in older women and often the masses themselves are highly attenuating because of hyalinisation. The regular shape and lack of invasive appearances indicate their benign nature.

Fa: fibroadenoma
Fl: fat island
SCF: subcutaneous fat

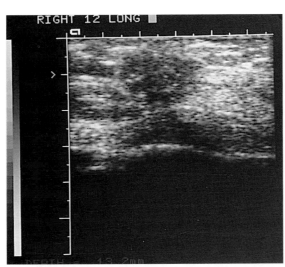 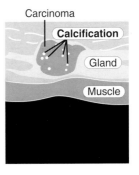

a

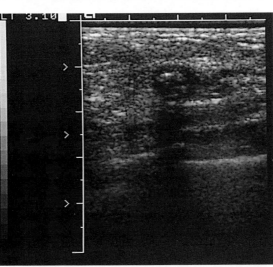 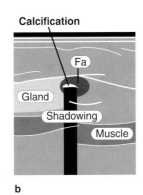

b

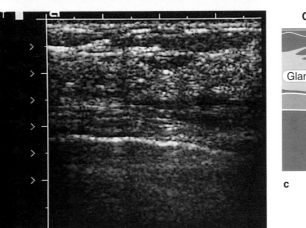 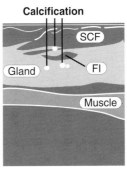

c

Cystic changes in tumours are not common but are occasionally seen in large malignancies with necrosis or haemorrhage (Fig. 4.7). Histologically, phylloides tumours and juvenile papillomatosis typically have cystic components, though these are uncommon types of tumour. Other conditions which often contain cystic areas are complex cysts, haematomas, abscesses and fat necrosis.

Intracystic tumours form a separate category, requiring special mention. Ultrasound is a very useful method to demonstrate solid portions of a predominantly cystic mass (Fig. 4.8)[3]; intraduct tumours, both papillomas and papillary carcinomas, may show this appearance. Ultrasound cannot differentiate between intraduct papillomas and non-invasive papillary carcinomas that remain confined within the duct, though the patient's age may provide a clue since intraductal papillomas tend to occur in a younger population than intracystic papillary carcinomas (see Ch. 5.3).

Fig. 4.7
Cystic change
This large lesion with a lobulated shape and posterior enhancement has very heterogeneous internal echoes, including some cystic regions. Cystic changes due to necrosis or bleeding are sometimes seen in large tumours.

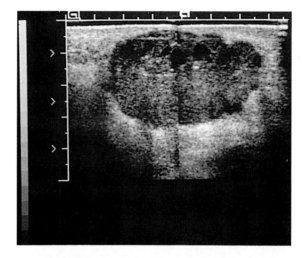
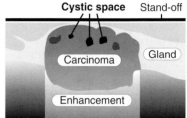

Fig. 4.8
Intracystic tumour
A solid nubbin is clearly seen within this cyst. The differential diagnosis lies between a papilloma and papillary carcinoma; they are usually indistinguishable on ultrasound.

DL: deep layer of the superficial fascia
GI: mammary gland
PE: posterior enhancement
SCF: subcutaneous fat
SL: superficial layer of the superficial fascia

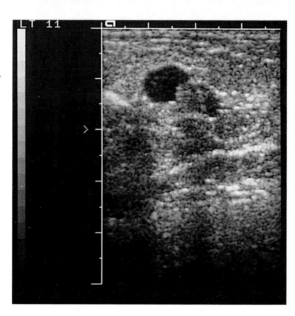
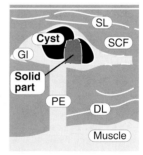

Intracystic echoes can also be caused by admixtures of different types of fluids. Echogenic fluid is confusing because it simulates soft tissue; its fluid nature may be suggested by a horizontal interface between the supernatant and dependent components and can be proved by observing particles in motion or gravitational settling on changing the patient's position (see Ch. 2). Bleeding within a cyst may also produce a fluid–fluid level due to separation of cells from serum; the serum is anechoic while the sediment returns low level echoes (Fig. 4.9). Spontaneous bleeding is highly suggestive of a proliferative lesion in the cyst wall (e.g. an intraductal papilloma or papillary carcinoma) even if the solid element is not separately identified.

The reverse pattern is seen in oil cysts due to fat necrosis: a horizontal interface delineates the surface between the echogenic supernatant fat and the anechoic dependent fluid layer (see Fig. 2.1). Milk of calcium, which is well seen on mediolateral mammograms, may also cause a fluid–fluid level but it is not commonly identified on ultrasound because the cysts that contain it are usually small and the scanty sediment is indistinguishable from the distal wall of the cyst (see Ch. 6.1).

Fig. 4.9
Intracystic echoes (fluid–fluid level)
Bleeding into a cyst may produce a fluid–fluid level. The dependent, echogenic portion (Fluid-2) contains cellular sediment, while the supernatant part (Fluid-1) is serous. Spontaneous bleeding into a cyst is highly suggestive of a proliferative lesion on the cyst wall, such as a papillary carcinoma or intraductal papilloma; in this case bleeding followed radiotherapy for an intracystic carcinoma.

ES: edge shadow

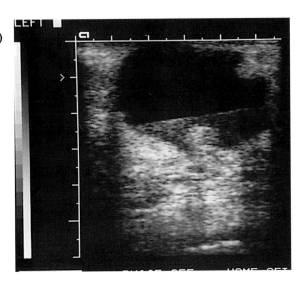
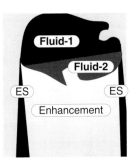

Edge and halo (boundary echoes)

The appearances of the margins of a mass can be classified according to their regularity and clarity of definition. The edge of a lesion may be regular or irregular, the former indicating a benign lesion, the latter usually suspicious of malignancy. However, edge irregularity is less apparent with some carcinomas and may be seen in some cases of benign mammary change that produce an infiltrating appearance, such as sclerosing adenosis or radial scars.

Perceived edge definition is determined by two factors.

One is the contrast of echo intensity between the mass and the surrounding tissues: if the lesion has a markedly different internal echo intensity than the surrounding tissues the edges tend to seem clear (Fig. 4.10.a), but if the internal echoes are similar to those of the surrounding tissues, the edges are indeterminate (Fig. 4.10.b). The other factor is gradient: where the echo intensity of the mass lesion changes gradually at the border, the edge is not clearly defined and a fuzzy margin results. This is typical of infiltrating lesions (Fig. 4.10.c) and of benign breast change.

Fig. 4.10
Edge definition
Edge definition is determined both by the contrast in reflectivity between the lesion and the surrounding tissues as well as by the rate of change of echo intensity across the edge (its gradient). Contrary to the usual pattern, carcinomas with very low internal echoes may have a clear margin (**a**), while a fibroadenoma whose echogenicity is similar to the surrounding tissues may have ill-defined margins (**b**). Highly invasive carcinomas usually have very ill-defined contours (**c**) because of their invading margins.

Ca: carcinoma
Fa: fibroadenoma
Gl: mammary gland
PE: posterior enhancement
RMS: retromammary space
SCF: subcutaneous fat
SL: superficial layer of the superficial fascia

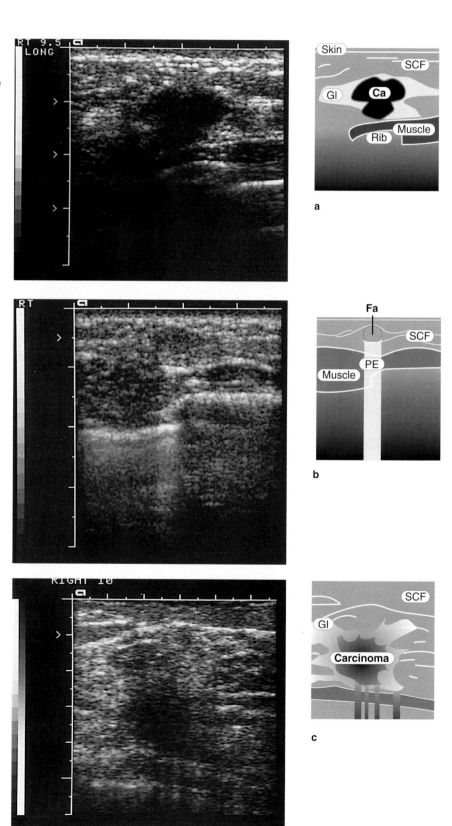

Edge shadows (Fig. 4.11) are caused by attenuation of the ultrasound beam at the lateral margins of the lesion and indicate that its edge is smooth (see description in Ch. 1). This sign has been emphasised as a benign feature but, in fact, any well-circumscribed lesion may produce edge shadows, whether benign or malignant. The same phenomenon occurs at the interface between different normal tissues, where it is sometimes called an 'interface shadow'; they are commonly seen behind Cooper's ligaments.

Fig. 4.11
Edge shadows
Edge shadows are produced by spreading of the ultrasonic beam at the vertical curvilinear smooth interface between differing tissues. This fibroadenoma has smooth margins which produce edge shadows that are well seen on both sides. They are emphasised by the high contrast with the enhancement produced by the lesion itself.

ES: edge shadow
Fa: fibroadenoma
Gl: mammary gland
PE: posterior enhancement

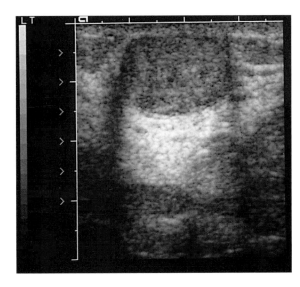

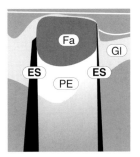

The halo (or boundary echo) is an ill-defined echogenic band at the surface of the lesion. It represents reflections from the invading margin around infiltrating malignancies and is commonly seen in carcinomas of the scirrhous type (Fig. 4.12.a). The alignment of the invading tissue strands across the ultrasound beam makes the halo more pronounced laterally than at the anterior surface (Fig. 4.13.a). Measurements should include the halo since this represents part of the tumour. Because of its origin, this appearance is almost specific for malignant lesions. Rarely, a halo may be produced by a non-malignant process where fibrosis extends into the surrounding breast tissue, such as in fat necrosis and postoperative scarring. Inflammatory processes extending around the lesion may cause a similar appearance with infected cysts or haematomas.

Strong echoes are commonly seen at the anterior surface of expanding lesions such as fibroadenomas (Fig. 4.13.b) and cysts; here they are usually attributable to the normal gland stretched over the lesion or, occasionally, to strong reflections from the smooth surface of the mass itself (Fig. 4.12.b). It is important not to confuse these well-defined, thin anterior echoes, which are common in benign lesions, with the echogenic lateral halo that indicates an invasive lesion and thus suggests malignancy.

Shadowing and enhancement

The intensity of the echoes deep to a lesion are determined by differences of attenuation between a lesion and the surrounding tissues (see Ch. 1). When a lesion attenuates more strongly, the deeper echoes are reduced in intensity causing 'shadowing', while lesions of low attenu-

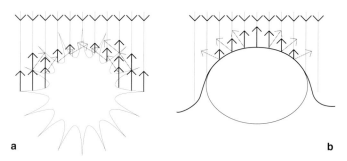

a   b

Fig. 4.12
Halo (boundary echoes)
A halo is produced by the reflections from the spiculated edge of a carcinoma. The halo is wider and more intense laterally (**a**) because the invading structures are aligned across the beam and so reflect more strongly. This suspicious halo must be distinguished from the echogenic rim often seen at the anterior surface of benign lesions with a smooth surface, here caused by the strong reflections from compressed normal tissues (**b**).

Fig. 4.13
Halo (boundary echoes)
A halo is typical of an invasive carcinoma (**a**). It is often seen in the scirrhous variety and, because of the rich fibrotic stroma typical of these tumours, it is usually accompanied by posterior shadows. Measurements of the tumour size should include the halo because this is part of the lesion. A thin, echogenic line may be seen at the anterior surface of a benign lesion (★**b**): this is a benign appearance, attributable to a compressed layer of normal tissue.

ES: edge shadow
Gl: mammary gland
Fa: fibroadenoma

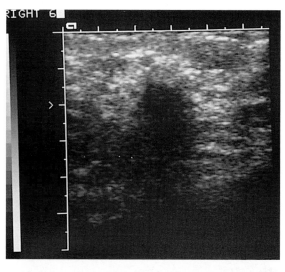

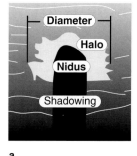

a

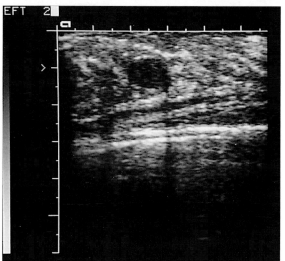

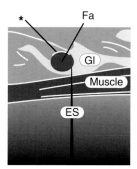

b

ation allow more sound to penetrate causing 'enhancement'. Where the attenuation in the lesion is the same as in the surrounding tissue, there is no change in the intensity of the deeper echoes. The degree of shadowing and enhancement may be classified as 'mild' or 'strong' by comparison with the surrounding echoes at the same depth.

Strong attenuation is a characteristic feature of breast carcinomas (Fig. 4.14.a); it was stressed as a reliable feature by the pioneers of breast echography. However, it is now generally accepted that some breast carcinomas do not produce any shadowing and, occasionally, they even show enhancement. Nevertheless, shadowing remains an important, if inconstant, sign of malignancy. The high attenuation is caused by the rich connective tissue stroma of many cancers[4] and so it is not surprising that scars, granulation tissues and hyalinised fibroadenomas may also cause shadowing.

Many pathologies do not affect attenuation and so produce neither shadowing nor enhancement (Fig. 4.14.b), while strong enhancement is a typical and diagnostic appearance of cysts (Fig. 4.14.c), of especial importance when they are small, where noise and reverberation artefacts make it difficult to be sure that there are no internal echoes. Many fibroadenomas also show enhancement, as do intracystic tumours.

Fig. 4.14
Shadowing and enhancement
a. Attenuative shadowing is a classical feature of carcinomas.
b. This fibroadenoma does not produce either shadowing or enhancement, a relatively rare pattern which may be encountered with both benign and malignant lesions.
c. Enhancement is typical of a cyst.

Ca: carcinoma
ES: edge shadow
Gl: mammary gland

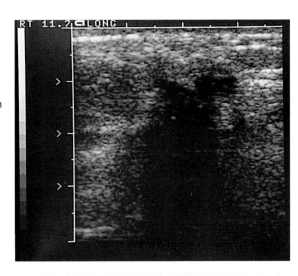
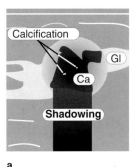

a

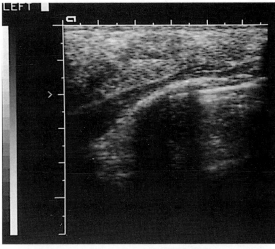
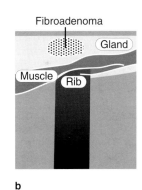

b

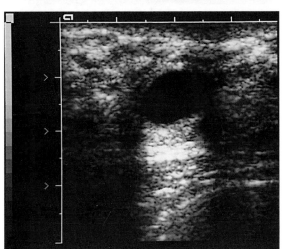
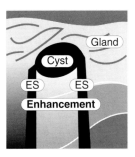

c

Secondary features

Invasion by a mass into the surrounding structures, together with reactive changes, produce secondary features which generally indicate malignancy. Since they are more apparent with larger, more obvious lesions, their practical value is in confirming the diagnosis and in evaluation of the extent of local invasion rather than in separating malignant from benign pathologies.

Interruption of adjacent structures
Carcinomas tend to invade as they grow, so they commonly interrupt surrounding structures (Fig. 4.15.a); by contrast, the expansile growth of benign lesions displaces adjacent normal tissues without disrupting them (Fig. 4.15.b). This feature is particularly useful in differentiating small carcinomas from benign masses[5]. On the other hand, when normal structures, such as ducts, can be demonstrated to run through an area of altered architecture, the abnormality is likely to be benign, most commonly due to benign breast change. Demonstration of these undisturbed ducts is particularly useful with lesions that contain sufficient fibrous tissue to produce shadowing, since this feature raises the possibility of malignancy (see Ch. 6.2).

Fig. 4.15
Interruption of adjacent structures
The superficial layer of the superficial fascia is interrupted in (**a**) (*arrow*) suggesting an invasive process (carcinoma); by contrast, the glandular tissue is smoothly stretched at the surface of the cyst (★) in (**b**).

Ca: carcinoma
DL: deep layer of the superficial fascia
Gl: mammary gland
RMS: retromammary space
SL: superficial layer of the superficial fascia

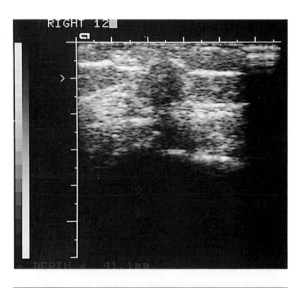

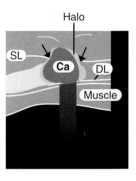

a

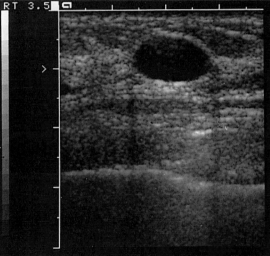

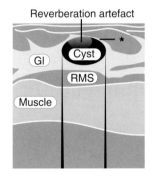

b

Duct dilatation

Localised duct dilatation may be observed with carcinomas, and may develop both peripherally and centrally due to obstruction (Fig. 4.16) or ductal spread, respectively. Echoes within the dilated ducts and irregularity or nodularity of the walls suggest ductal invasion or an intraductal papilloma or carcinoma; here the dilatation usually results from bleeding from the fragile surfaces of the tumour.

Skin thickening

Skin thickening can be caused either by direct invasion by a carcinoma (Fig. 4.17.a), or by oedema, either inflammatory or due to lymphatic occlusion (Fig. 4.17.b). It is a typical feature of inflammatory carcinomas but is also encountered in infective mastitis.

Fig. 4.16
Duct dilatation
A duct obstructed by a carcinoma is dilated peripherally. Note the lateral halo and the lack of distal shadowing from this 15 mm carcinoma.

Ca: carcinoma
Gl: mammary gland
SCF: superficial layer of the superficial fascia

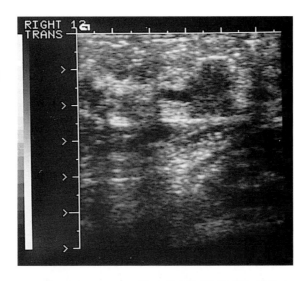
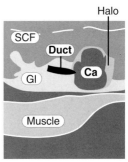

Fig. 4.17
Skin thickening
a. The skin may be thickened by direct malignant invasion. In this carcinoma, the area of the skin thickening is more extensive than the area of direct invasion.
b. Skin thickening is a common feature of inflammatory carcinomas. Dilated lymphatics may also be seen beneath the skin.

RMS: retromammary space
SCF: subcutaneous fat

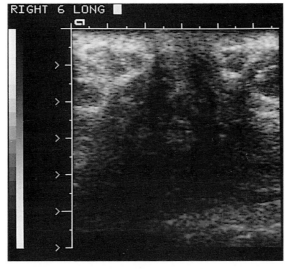
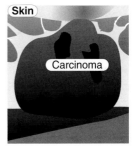

a

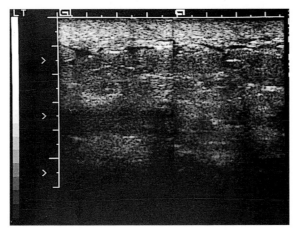
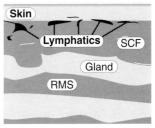

b

Echogenicity of the subcutaneous fat

In highly infiltrative carcinomas, the echogenicity of the subcutaneous fatty tissue may be increased (Fig. 4.18). The change is probably due to oedema following tumour invasion into lymphatics and may be focal or diffuse. Skin oedema often coexists; it produces the peau d'orange appearance. The change in echogenicity is most easily assessed by comparison with the opposite breast, especially when the process is diffuse, in which case it is easily overlooked completely. Increased echogenicity of the subcutaneous fat may also be observed in inflammatory processes, including traumatic lesions and following radiotherapy. The exact mechanism of the increase in echogenicity of fat in these circumstances is a matter of debate: an increase in fluid in other organs, such as the kidney or liver, usually decreases their echogenicity. It may be that this occurs in an already fluid-rich organ because the interfaces are separated out, whereas fluid added to a fatty tissue increases its echogenicity by increasing the number of fat/fluid interfaces which are strong reflectors of ultrasound.

Venous and lymphatic dilatation

Tubular structures are occasionally observed in advanced carcinomas, especially in cases with diffusely increased subcutaneous fat echoes. Where they are due to dilated arteries, the blood flow is easily demonstrated on a colour Doppler study (described later in this chapter), but the arteries of neoplasms are difficult to identify on conventional images because they are small. Arteries dilate in pregnancy and lactation, and are occasionally detected in apparently healthy older patients — presumably these are atherosclerotic vessels. Veins may also dilate in association with breast carcinomas; they are usually observed immediately under the skin (Fig. 4.19, Plate C.7.b). Veins are easily compressed by the pressure of the transducer, so a light touch is required to detect them. By contrast, lymphatics are only visible when they are obstructed, and so they are less compressible. Additional points of distinction are that lymphatics lie deeper in the breast and do not give Doppler signals. Situations that lead to dilated vessels are often also responsible for skin thickening and increased subcutaneous fat echoes. The causes are listed in Table 4.2.

Fig. 4.18
Carcinoma with echogenic subcutaneous fat
This highly infiltrative carcinoma has caused increased echogenicity of the fatty tissue at its surface, due to focal lymphoedema. Lymphatic invasion was found on histology.

Ca: carcinoma
Gl: mammary gland
LE: increased subcutaneous echoes due to lymphatic oedema
SCF: subcutaneous fat

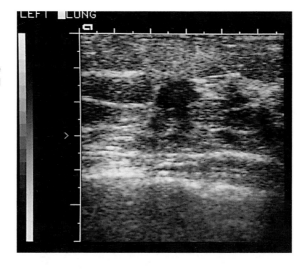
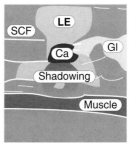

Table 4.2   Causes and appearances of dilated vessels in the breast

	Appearances	Causes
Lymphatic congestion	Dilated lymphatics Skin thickening	Axillary lymphatic obstruction (a) Extensive nodal metastasis from breast carcinomas or primary lymphatic diseases (e.g. lymphoma, leukaemia) (b) Mediastinal tumour or lymphadenopathy, anterior chest wall tumour, advanced pelvic malignancy* (as a collateral lymphatic flow)
	Increased echogenicity of subcutaneous fat	Postoperative, postirradiation
Venous congestion	Dilated veins Skin thickening Increased echogenicity of subcutaneous fat	Right heart failure Generalised fluid retention
Arterial supply increased	Dilated veins Increased arterial flow especially on colour Doppler (Increased echogenicity of subcutaneous fat) (Skin thickening)	Pregnancy, lactation Carcinoma Inflammation, infection, trauma, irradiation

* Lymphoedema of the breast due to pelvic malignancy is reported on mammography.

Fig. 4.19
Venous dilatation
Dilatation of a subcutaneous vein seen in an advanced breast carcinoma. Veins are often seen parallel to the skin and are compressible.

SCF: subcutaneous fat
SL: superficial layer of the superficial fascia

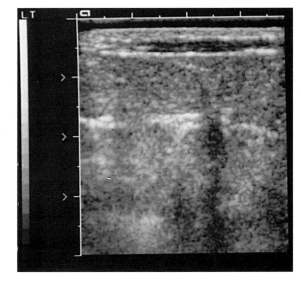
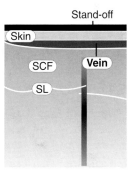

Lymph node enlargement

The commonest site for lymph node metastases is the axilla. Although benign lymph nodes are often palpable and can be demonstrated on mammograms (Fig. 4.20.a), they are hardly ever detected on ultrasound. This is because they are buried in fatty tissue which has the same echogenicity. Oval structures with an echogenic centre (corresponding to the hilar fat or vessels) are the typical appearances of normal or enlarged benign lymph nodes (Fig. 4.20.b), though microscopic metastasis cannot be excluded. Lymph nodes containing gross metastases are much easier to detect: they are seen as relatively well-cir-cumscribed rounded, lobulated or slightly irregular structures, often multiple, with homogeneous but obviously lower internal echoes than the surrounding fatty tissues (Fig. 4.20c). The limited resolution of ultrasound means that microscopic metastatic nodal involvement cannot be detected or excluded.

Normal lymph nodes lying high in the axilla (levels II and III) and in the parasternal, intermuscular (Rotter) or supraclavicular regions, are not visualised on ultrasound; if detected, they are always pathological and usually contain metastatic tumour.

Fig. 4.20
Axillary lymph node
Axillary lymph nodes are commonly seen on mammograms in normal subjects (**a**). They often contain a radiolucent hilum, representing fat deposited in the hilum. On ultrasound (**b**) the reflectivity of the lymph node is very similar to that of the surrounding fat, while the echogenic hilum is similar to the connective tissues in the surrounding tissues; normal axillary lymph nodes are therefore difficult to demonstrate. However, those enlarged by metastatic involvement are much more readily detected (**c**) being seen as echo-poor masses. They are round or lobulated rather than the oval shape of a normal or reactive lymph node.

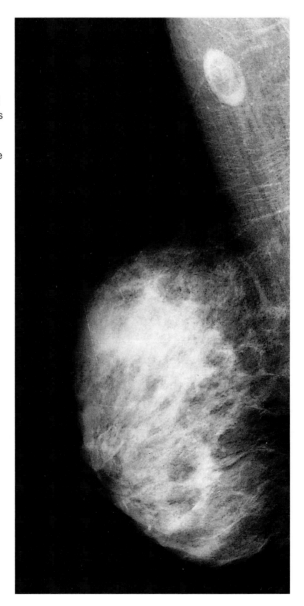

a

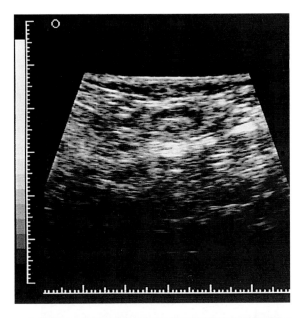

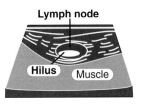

b

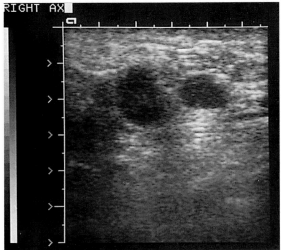

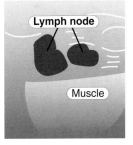

c

Intramammary lymph nodes are sometimes demonstrated on mammograms that are otherwise normal and have been reported in up to 28% of breasts with carcinomas[6]. Benign intramammary lymph nodes have a characteristic mammographic appearance with a lucent centre or hilar notch; they are usually small (<1 cm) and impalpable. They are difficult to identify on ultrasound, not only because of their small size, but also because they usually have almost the same echogenicity as fatty tissue, while the hilar structures are similar in appearance to the fibrous tissue seen elsewhere in the breast. Occasionally, a palpable lump can be diagnosed as an intramammary lymph node on ultrasound by its characteristic features: an oval, isoechoic or slightly echo-poor nodule (compared with the fatty tissue) with an echogenic line representing the hilum (Fig. 4.21.a)[7].

Metastatic intramammary lymph nodes are larger and so are more easily detected. They are usually round, well-circumscribed and less echogenic than benign nodes (Fig. 4.21.b). Differentiation from coexisting benign masses, intraductal spread from the primary tumour or a second primary is difficult because lymph nodes containing metastases usually lose their morphological characteristics and the hilum is obliterated.

Dynamic tests

The response of normal and pathological tissues to attempts at compression and displacement as observed on real-time form additional diagnostic features that are especially useful in equivocal cases[8]. The lesion may be manipulated directly with the free hand, or with the transducer (see Ch. 2).

Compressibility

Most malignancies are incompressible, a feature that is particularly useful in the diagnosis of well-circumscribed carcinomas which may simulate benign lesions and in those with the same reflectivity as the surrounding tissues ('isoechoic' lesions), which are all too easily overlooked entirely. Cysts are usually compressible, a feature that is reassuring when the ultrasound appearances are complex, though rounded, tense cysts are occasionally encountered. Fibroadenomas are usually somewhat compressible though, when calcified or hyalinised, they can also be hard and incompressible. Benign breast change sometimes forms a localised echo-poor region which is difficult to differentiate from malignancy because of its irregular shape and ill-defined margins. However, these areas are usually at least partly compressible and this feature may be the only indicator of its benign nature.

Fig. 4.21
Intramammary lymph nodes
a. This mass in the axillary tail of the left breast has the typical appearance of a lymph node: an oval nodule with echogenic centre. Benign intramammary lymph nodes are very difficult to detect unless they are first located by palpation.
b. Metastatic intramammary lymph node. This woman presented with extensive lymphadenopathy. The two breast nodules shown were presumed to be additional involved lymph nodes but on histology an intraductal component was found in one, indicating that this was the primary. The smaller was an intramammary node containing breast carcinoma cells.

Ca: carcinoma
Gl: mammary gland

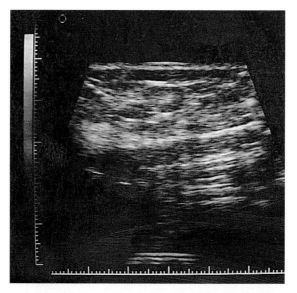
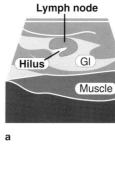
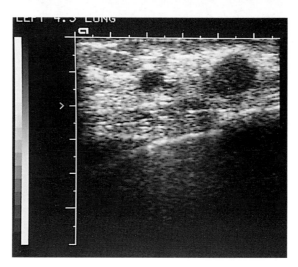
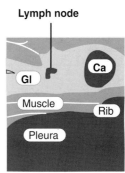

The behaviour under compression is also useful for differentiation between benign and malignant shadows. Shadowing that disappears when the tissue is compressed by the transducer is usually benign, whereas shadowing from a schirrous carcinoma cannot be obliterated by probe pressure. Care should be taken to ensure that the lesion remains in the slice plane during compression to avoid mistaking apparent loss of shadowing for sideways movement of the lesion out of the field of view.

Mobility

Carcinomas tend to be locally fixed because of invasion into the surrounding tissues. The echogenic halo is often more obvious when the lesion is moved than on the frozen image. Fibroadenomas are typically very mobile, even those that are calcified or hyalinised when their heterogeneous internal echoes and posterior shadowing may suggest malignancy. Cysts and focal regions of benign mammary change are relatively immobile since they form part of the ductal structures of the breast, though typically they are moderately compressible.

In advanced carcinomas, exclusion of fixation to the muscular layer by demonstrating mobility on real-time scanning is useful in preoperative evaluation or as a guide to appropriate therapy.

Doppler features

A simple use of Doppler depends on the fact that fluid spaces are never vascular. Thus the demonstration of blood flow within a lesion excludes a cyst (either complex or simple), galactocele, haematoma or an abscess cavity.

A more sophisticated application is the discrimination between carcinomas and benign breast disorders, in which the initial enthusiastic reports[9] have been tempered by the overlap found in subsequent studies. The main differentiating feature is vascular density[10], especially when related to the size of the lesion. Increased flow within the lesion and at its margin is usually seen in breast carcinomas (Plate C.7.a), even those as small as 1 cm in diameter, though generally the smaller the lesion, the less obvious the flow. Doppler signals may not always be detected

in very small or in situ carcinomas. Doppler is particularly useful as an indicator of malignancy in well-circumscribed tumours which may have benign appearances (Plate C.7.b). Occasionally a lesion is first detected by its colour Doppler signals, especially in a large breast (Plate C.7.c).

Tumour vessels are typically tortuous, unlike the relatively straight normal vessels of the breast, and they lie within or at the margins of the mass, whereas normal vessels tend to run along the anterior surface of the gland or along the Cooper's ligaments. The Doppler signals are strong (high amplitude), the flow velocity is high while a low resistance pattern with continued flow in diastole is seen on the spectral tracing[11]. Pulsatile venous flow of high velocity may also be seen, and is probably due to the arteriovenous shunts that are typical of tumour vessels.

Undetectable or scanty flow is typical of benign breast change (Plate C.8) and fibroadenomas (Plate C.9). Large benign tumours, especially phylloides tumours and fibroadenomas in young women, sometimes show increased numbers of vessels (Plate C.10) and, very occasionally, no vessels can be detected in breast carcinomas, even of moderate size, so that there is some overlap in the Doppler findings. The Doppler features probably relate to the proliferative activity of the lesion.

Inflammatory lesions are an exception: they often have very marked flow with an increase both of vessel density and flow velocity. Doppler studies are often negative in treated carcinomas and recurrences.

The reported incidences of the ultrasound findings in breast malignancies (almost all primary carcinomas) are listed in Table 4.3.

Table 4.3 Ultrasound features of malignant lesions						
	Hackelöer[12] N=200	Harper[13] N=41	Egan[14] N=107	Cole-Beuglet[15] N=80	Leucht[16] N=353	Vlaisavljevic[17] N=84
Shape						
Irregular	–	–	–	–	–	63%
Internal echoes						
Weak	–	–	–	84%	56%*	–
Heterogeneous	66%	70%	70%	–	89%	39%
Edge						
Irregular	–	88%	86%	72%	93%	–
Ill-defined	84%	–	–	–	94%	–
Posterior echoes						
Shadowing	74%	97%	73%	90%	44%**	39%
Dynamic tests						
Incompressibility	–	–	–	–	72%	–

* Internal echoes classified as 'very low' ('low' internal echoes excluded).
** Unilateral shadows excluded.

DISORDERS WITHOUT A MASS

Between 5 and 10% of breast carcinomas do not produce a mass that can be identified on ultrasound—some being completely undetected, others causing only minor architectural disturbances[15,18]. Breast diseases that may not form a mass are listed in Table 4.4. They are difficult or even impossible to diagnose on ultrasound.

Benign breast change does not usually form a distinct mass but produces textural changes which are usually diffuse and bilateral but may be focal (Fig. 4.22.a). Intraductal carcinomas usually cannot be detected on ultrasound, but, if extensive, they may cause focal textural changes with a very similar pattern to focal benign breast change. Some invasive carcinomas, especially the infiltrating lobular type, may produce only textural distortion (Fig. 4.22.b) or extensive shadowing without either a definite mass or reactive changes, even when the lesion is large. The ultrasound appearances are confusingly similar to those of severe benign breast change, particularly in cases with marked fibrosis, especially when there are no secondary features of malignancy.

Table 4.4 Disorders without a mass	
Benign	**Malignant**
Benign mammary change	Intraductal carcinoma, especially comedo type
Inflammation without abscess formation	Some invasive carcinomas, especially infiltrating lobular carcinoma
Irradiated breast	
	Inflammatory carcinoma

Mastitis is not common except during lactation where the history is typical and further investigation is not needed. However, the ultrasound features such as skin thickening and the increased echogenicity of the subcutaneous tissues are very similar to those of an inflammatory carcinoma, though here the changes are more severe. Similar changes may occur following irradiation.

Fig. 4.22
Focal architectural change
a. In this case an echo-poor area was seen at the site of extensive microcalcification on the mammogram. On histology of the excision biopsy, only benign mammary change was found.
b. Only textural distortion with some shadowing could be demonstrated at the site of a hard mass which was clinically a carcinoma. On histology an invasive lobular carcinoma was found.

GI: mammary gland
SCF: subcutaneous fat

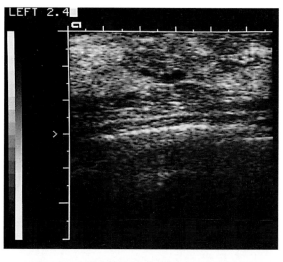
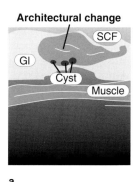

a

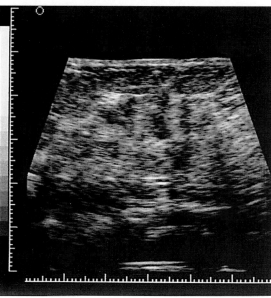
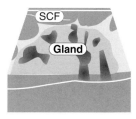

b

REFERENCES

1. T. Tajima, M. Kubota, T. Mitomi et al: Longitudinal/transverse ratio of tumor echogram as a diagnostic criterion of breast carcinoma. In: Ultrasonic Examination of the Breast, edited by J. Jellins and T. Kobayashi. John Wiley, 1983, pp 69–70.
2. F. Kasumi, H. Tanaka: Detection of microcalcifications in breast carcinoma by ultrasound. In: Ultrasonic Examination of the Breast, edited by J. Jellins and T. Kobayashi. John Wiley, 1983, pp 89–97.
3. K. Reuter, C.J. D'Orsi, F. Reale: Intracystic carcinoma of the breast: the role of ultrasonography. Radiology 153; 233–234, 1984.
4. T. Kobayashi: Diagnostic ultrasound in breast cancer: analysis of retrotumorous echo patterns correlated with sonic attenuation by cancerous connective tissue. J. Clin Ultrasound 7; 471–479, 1979.
5. Y. Konishi, M. Ogata, T. Kuroki, et al: Assessment on differential diagnosis between tumor-forming mastopathy on ultrasonography and T1 breast cancer. Jpn J Med Ultrasonics 15; 420–428, 1988.
6. R.L. Egan, M.B. McSweeney: Intramammary lymph nodes. Cancer 51; 1838–1842, 1983.
7. P.B. Gordon, B. Gilks: Sonographic appearance of normal intramammary lymph nodes. J Ultrasound Med 7; 545–548, 1988.
8. E. Ueno, E. Tohno, S. Soeda et al: Dynamic tests in real-time breast echography. Ultrasound Med Biol 14 (suppl 1) 53–57, 1988.
9. S.G. Schoenberger, C.M. Sutherland, A.E. Robinson: Breast neoplasms: duplex sonographic imaging as an adjunct in diagnosis. Radiology 168; 665–668, 1988.
10. D.O. Cosgrove, J.C. Bamber, J.B. Davey et al: Colour Doppler signals from breast tumours. Radiology 176; 175–180, 1990.
11. P.N. Burns, J.D. Davies, M. Halliwell, et al: Doppler ultrasound in the diagnosis of breast cancer. In: Ultrasound in Breast and Endocrine Disease — Clinics in Diagnostic Ultrasound (12), edited by G.R. Leopold. Churchill Livingstone, New York, 1984, pp 41–56.
12. B.-J. Hackelöer, V. Duda, G. Lauth: Ultrasound Mammography. Springer-Verlag, New York, 1989.
13. A.P. Harper, E. Kelly-Fry, J.S. Noe, et al: Ultrasound in the evaluation of solid breast masses. Radiology 146; 731–736, 1983.
14. R.L. Egan, K.L. Egan: Automated water-path full-breast sonography: correlation with histology of 176 solid lesions. AJR 143; 499–507, 1984.
15. C. Cole-Beuglet, R.Z. Soriano, A.B. Kurtz, B.B. Goldberg: Ultrasound analysis of 104 primary breast carcinomas classified according to histopathologic type. Radiology 147; 191–196, 1983.
16. W.J. Leucht, D.R. Rabe, K.D. Humbert: Diagnostic value of interpretative criteria in real-time sonography of the breast. Ultrasound Med Biol 14 (suppl 1); 59–73, 1988.
17. V. Vlaisavljevic: Differentiation of solid breast tumors on the basis of their primary echographic characteristics as revealed by real-time scanning of the uncompressed breast. Ultrasound Med Biol 14 (suppl 1); 59–73, 1988.
18. D.B. Kopans, J.E. Meyer, R.T. Steinbock: Breast cancer: the appearances as delineated by whole breast water-bath ultrasound scanning. J Clin Ultrasound 10; 313–322, 1982.

Chapter 5

Benign processes – tumours

5.1 FIBROADENOMA

CLINICAL FEATURES

Fibroadenomas are very common tumours, occurring at any age in premenopausal women (15–50 years), but more commonly in the young. Fibroadenomas do not usually appear for the first time or grow after the menopause except in women taking hormone replacement therapy (HRT)[1] but they may persist and are sometimes found incidentally on mammography or ultrasound in the involuted breast. Many of these incidental lesions are impalpable; ultrasound is useful to localise them, to determine their internal structures and especially to differentiate them from cysts. Fibroadenomas may grow rapidly during pregnancy and they occasionally undergo spontaneous infarction or necrosis without any symptoms. Fibroadenomas are commonly multiple (Fig. 5.1) and they may be bilateral.

On palpation, they are rounded, ovoid or lobulated masses and are usually firm or rubbery in consistency. If they calcify they can become hard. Their relative mobility in the breast tissue is a characteristic feature; for this reason fibroadenomas are commonly known as 'breast mice'.

Carcinoma arising within a fibroadenoma is rare; when it occurs it is usually of the in situ lobular type[2].

PATHOLOGICAL FEATURES

Fibroadenomas are circumscribed lesions composed of fibrous and epithelial elements. They may have a thin capsule or abut directly on the surrounding tissue. Two types of growth pattern have been observed: pericanalicular and intracanalicular. In the former, the epithelial component consists of rounded duct-like structures that retain their shape and are surrounded by stroma, often with a concentric arrangement. In the latter, stromal overgrowth results in considerable elongation, thinning and distortion of the epithelial elements, often with obliteration of the lumina. Although fibroadenomas have been classified according to these growth patterns, there is no evidence of any difference in behaviour and both patterns may be seen in the same lesion (Plate P.5.1).

Most of the epithelium in fibroadenomas is derived from the terminal duct lobular units and consequently may undergo the physiological and pathological changes typical of these structures. Thus, secretory changes are seen in pregnancy and lactation while cysts, adenosis, hyperplasia and even in situ carcinoma may occur, usually when these changes are also present in the surrounding breast.

The stromal components vary in appearance, particularly in cellularity. Less cellular lesions tend to occur in older subjects and occasionally they may be completely hyalinised and partly calcified. More cellular tumours usually occur in younger subjects and often exhibit myxoid change; the term 'juvenile fibroadenoma' is sometimes used to describe highly cellular, rapidly growing tumours in adolescents (Plate P.5.2). Care should be taken to distinguish the more cellular examples from low grade phylloides tumours, particularly if they occur in older subjects.

The stroma of fibroadenomas is usually entirely fibroblastic but adipose tissue and smooth muscle may be seen occasionally. Foci of cartilage and bone are very rarely observed.

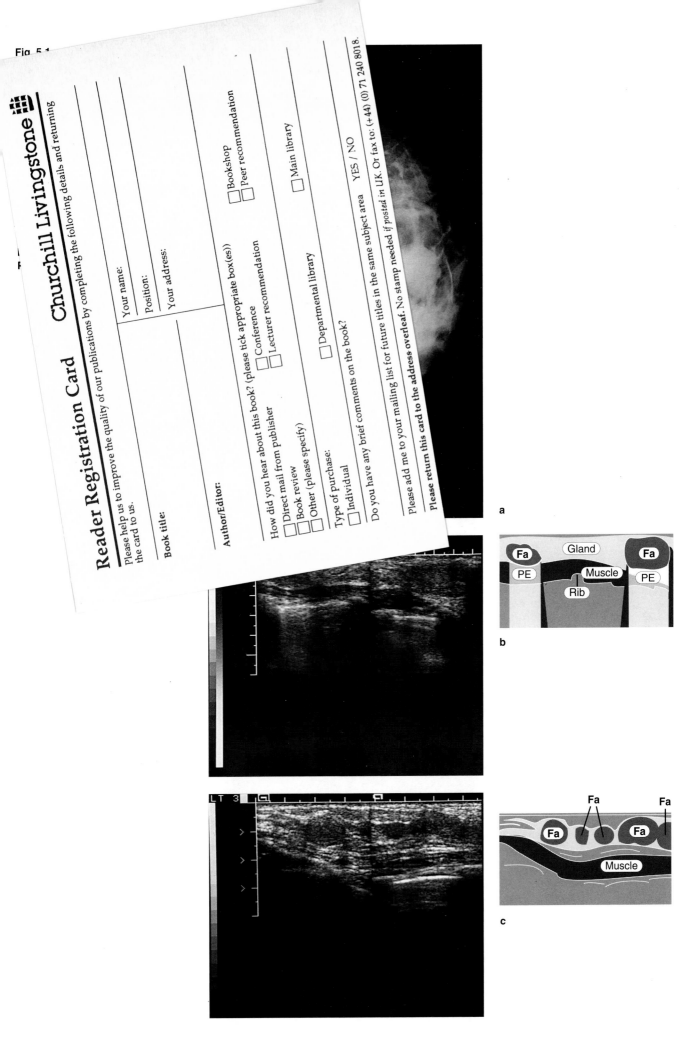

a

b

Fa Gland Fa
PE Muscle PE
Rib

c

Fa   Fa
Fa Fa
Muscle

ULTRASOUND FEATURES

The appearances are variable[3], but regularity of structure and lack of invasion are critical to the diagnosis. Examples of typical fibroadenomas are shown in Fig. 5.2.

Fig. 5.2
Typical fibroadenomas
a. An oval shape and smooth, well-defined margins with a uniform echo texture and bilateral edge shadows are the classical appearances of a fibroadenoma.
b. Another typical fibroadenoma with an oval shape and posterior enhancement.
c. This oval mass with posterior enhancement is a typical fibroadenoma. The internal texture is coarse but uniform. The glandular layer at the surface of this mass is smoothly compressed.

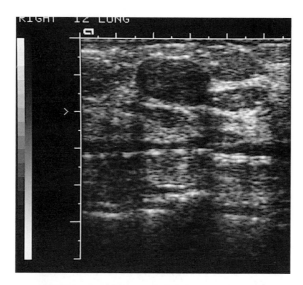

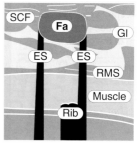

a

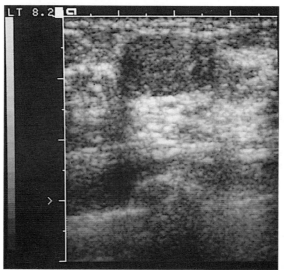

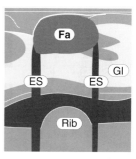

b

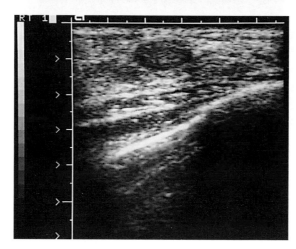

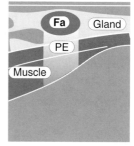

c

d. This fibroadenoma has relatively strong echoes and the internal texture is grainy but uniform. The edge shadows indicate a smooth contour.

e. A fibroadenoma in a thin breast. The oval shape of this mass indicates that it is non-invasive. The texture is homogeneous. (Reverberation artefacts are seen because of the strong reflections between the muscular surface of the rib and the transducer.

f. This fibroadenoma is small and almost spherical in shape because it has a firm consistency. There is a slight indentation of the muscular surface. However, its margin is smooth and there are no signs of invasion.

ES: edge shadow
Fa: fibroadenoma
Gl: mammary gland
PE: posterior enhancement
RMS: retromammary space
SCF: subcutaneous fat

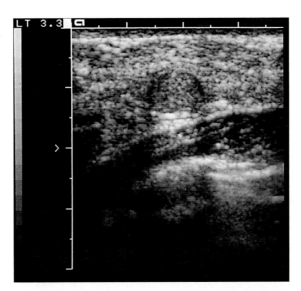

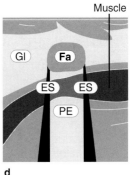

d

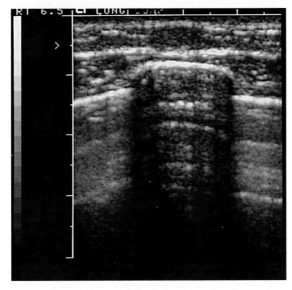

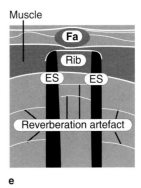

e

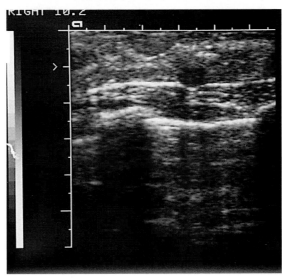

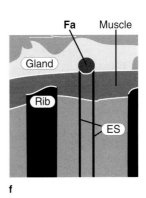

f

The majority of fibroadenomas have an oval shape in which the AP diameter (depth) is less than the transverse diameter (width)[4] (Fig. 5.3). Although many authors describe fibroadenomas as rounded in shape[5,6], with hand-held real-time scans and the patient supine, fibroadenomas that are completely spherical (i.e. those with a D:W ratio of 1.0) are rarely encountered except in small lesions (<1 cm). It is extremely rare to encounter a fibroadenoma in which the AP diameter is larger than the width because fibroadenomas are usually soft and can be flattened even by slight pressure of the transducer. Furthermore, fibroadenomas are mobile and tend to become orientated along rather than across the ductal elements. Sometimes fibroadenomas have small notches or a lobulated shape (Fig. 5.4).

Fig. 5.3
The D:W (depth:width) ratio
The D:W ratio of this fibroadenoma is about 0.5 (0.8 cm × 1.5 cm). Fibroadenomas usually lie flat with the patient supine and the depth:width ratio is less than 1.0 and usually below 0.8.

SCF: subcutaneous fat
Fa: fibroadenoma
Gl: mammary gland
PE: posterior enhancement

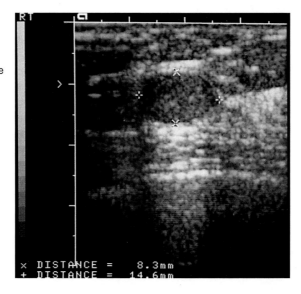

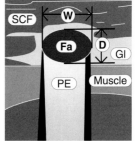

Fig. 5.4
Lobulated fibroadenomas
a. Fibroadenomas often have a slightly lobulated shape. Note the notch at the anterior surface of this example.
b. Marked lobulation, as in this fibroadenoma, is unusual; the differential diagnosis is a phylloides tumour. Histologically this was a fibroadenoma.
c. This 4 cm mass also has a lobulated shape with well-circumscribed margins (note the slightly echogenic rim, due to compressed overlying gland). It has a homogeneous texture, though there are some echogenic lines which are probably due to fibrous strands. Histologically this was a fibroadenoma.

Fa: fibroadenoma
Gl: mammary gland
PE: posterior enhancement

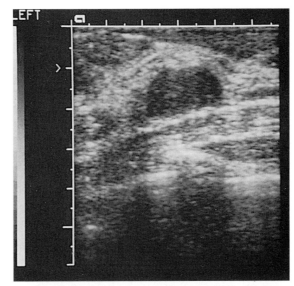
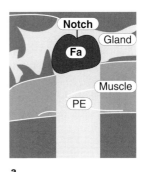

a

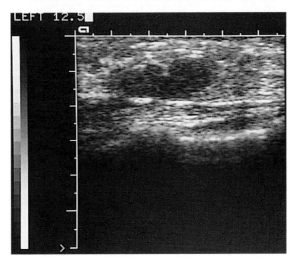
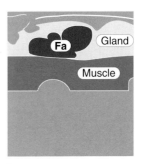

b

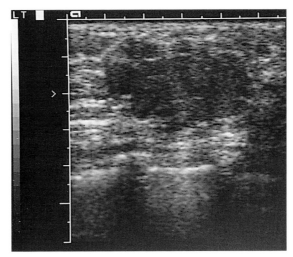
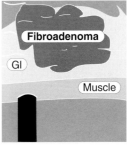

c

The echo intensity of fibroadenomas is variable; usually their echoes are 'very low', 'low', or 'equal to fatty tissue' (Fig. 5.5) and occasionally they have echoes 'stronger than fatty tissue'. Slightly echo-poor lesions (less reflective than fat) are commonest and fibroadenomas are generally more reflective than cancers. When the internal echoes are equal to those from the surrounding fatty tissue, fibroadenomas are difficult to distinguish from fat lobules, especially on static images. This is the commonest cause of failure to visualise a fibroadenoma on ultrasound, a problem affecting up to 14% of cases studied with static scanners[3,6]. Failure to detect fibroade-

nomas is less of a problem with real-time scanners (about 1%)[4]. By contrast, carcinomas with the same echogenicity as fat are rare.

Fig. 5.5
Internal echoes of fibroadenomas
a. A fibroadenoma with very low internal echoes.

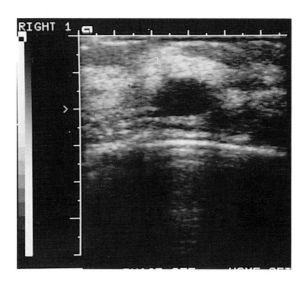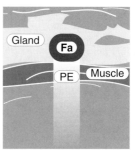

a

b. This fibroadenoma has slightly lower echogenicity than the fatty tissue. This is the commonest pattern.
c. Fibroadenoma with echoes of almost the same intensity as the surrounding fat. This type is often missed on static scanning or if the lesion is impalpable because of its similarity to fat lobules, though these do not usually have posterior enhancement, as this fibroadenoma shows.

Fa: fibroadenoma
PE: posterior enhancement.

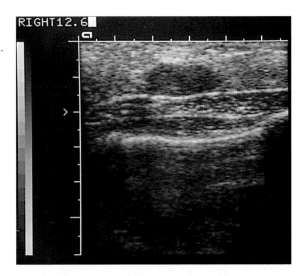

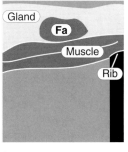

b

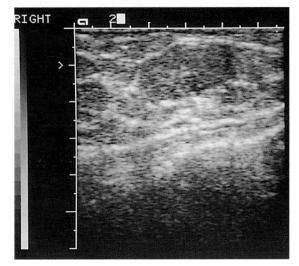

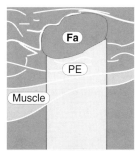

c

The internal echo of a fibroadenoma is usually homogeneous with a somewhat coarse or grainy texture. There is no difference on ultrasound between the two types of growth pattern — pericanalicular and intracanalicular. If calcification occurs, the lesion becomes heterogeneous. Although cystic spaces may be seen on histology as 'clefts', they are rarely detected on ultrasound and, if present, the possibility of a phylloides tumour must be kept in mind. 'Cystic change' may also be seen after aspiration cytology, here actually representing haemorrhage.

Calcification tends to occur in older patients. The foci are usually large enough to cause shadowing as well as strong echoes (Fig. 5.6).

Fig. 5.6
Fibroadenomas with calcification
a. The coarse calcification in a fibroadenoma is seen as bright echoes with shadowing. It also produces a heterogeneous internal texture. In this example there is also posterior shadowing because this is an old and probably hyalinised lesion. Its lobulated but smooth margin without invasion indicates a fibroadenoma. Demonstrating mobility on dynamic tests is also helpful to rule out malignancy in this type of lesion.
b. The mammogram of the fibroadenoma in (**a**) shows coarse flecks of calcification.

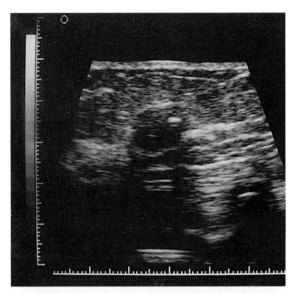
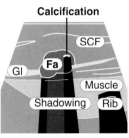

a

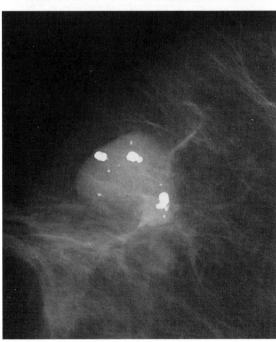

b

c. A heavily calcified fibroadenoma shows curvilinear strong surface echoes with marked shadowing which prevents an assessment of the shape or the texture of the lesion. This type of calcification may be seen in calcified cysts and lymph nodes: it indicates a benign process. Another fibroadenoma (non-calcified) is seen in the same scan.

d. The mammogram of this lesion (**c**) shows that it is almost totally calcified.

Fa: fibroadenoma
Gl: mammary gland
SCF: subcutaneous fat

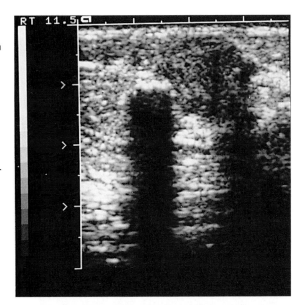

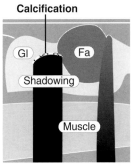

c

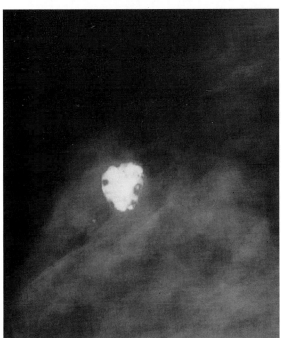

d

Most commonly, fibroadenomas are well-circumscribed and have smooth, sharp margins. However, lesions with relatively strong internal echoes may seem to have fuzzy contours because of the low contrast with the surrounding tissues (Fig. 5.7). Fibroadenomas do not have a halo (boundary echoes) in the true meaning of the term, though their anterior margins can seem brighter because of the stretched overlying layer of normal tissue (Fig. 5.8). This feature indicates expansile growth rather than invasion. Because the margins are sharp and smooth, edge shadows (interface shadows) are usually present; they are caused by refraction and beam spreading and do not have the same suspicious implications as attenuative shadowing.

The posterior echoes may be enhanced (the commonest pattern) or show no change; occasionally, in calcified or hyalinised lesions, there may be shadowing (Fig. 5.9). Fibroadenomas in young patients tend to show marked enhancement because of their rich cellularity and paucity of fibrous tissue.

Fig. 5.7
Fibroadenoma with ill-defined margins
This mass has relatively strong internal echoes and its margins are ill-defined. However, the oval shape and homogeneous internal echoes are typical appearances of a fibroadenoma. The edge shadows also indicate that it has smooth margins.

ES: edge shadow
Fa: fibroadenoma
PE: posterior enhancement

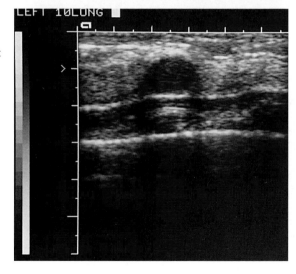

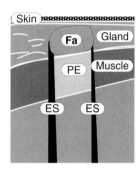

Fig. 5.8
A fibroadenoma with an echogenic anterior margin
A curvilinear echogenic line is seen at the anterior surface of this fibroadenoma (★). It is due to strong reflections from a stretched layer of glandular tissue and must be differentiated from the lateral halo typical of a carcinoma. The margin border of this fibroadenoma has produced edge shadows.

ES: edge shadow
Fa: fibroadenoma
PE: posterior enhancement

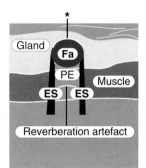

Fig. 5.9

Distal echoes in fibroadenomas

a. Fibroadenomas usually produce distal enhancement which contrasts strongly with the typical edge shadows.

b. Fibroadenomas sometimes have no enhancement, as in this example. An echogenic rim at the anterior surface is compressed glandular tissue, indicating expansile rather than invasive growth.

c. Fibroadenoma with posterior attenuation. This rare type is easily misdiagnosed as a carcinoma. However, this lesion has a thin echogenic rim and a lobulated but regular shape. Histologically it proved to be a hyalinised fibroadenoma.

DL: deep layer of the superficial fascia
ES: edge shadow
Fa: fibroadenoma
Gl: mammary gland
PE: posterior enhancement
SL: superficial layer of the superficial fascia

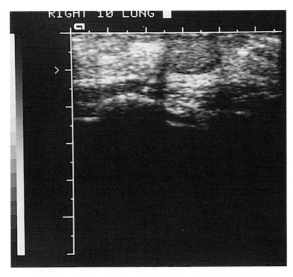
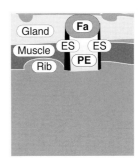

a

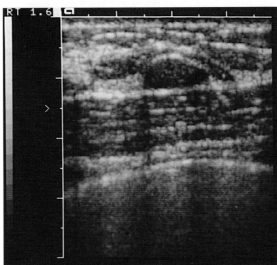
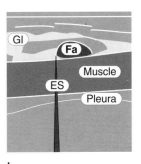

b

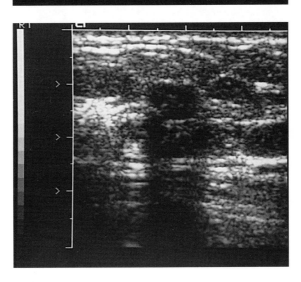
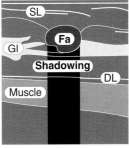

c

An important clinical characteristic of fibroadenomas is their mobility; this is equally apparent on ultrasound. The masses slip between the surrounding tissue and even revolve under gentle pressure (Fig. 5.10). These features are very important in making the correct diagnosis especially with atypical lesions such as those that shadow, those with a heterogeneous texture and those containing calcification. Fibroadenomas are usually relatively incompressible (Fig. 5.11), a feature that may suggest malignancy, though the mobility of a fibroadenoma is obviously different from the fixation of malignant masses. Fibroadenomas are never attached to the pectoral fascia or skin.

The majority of fibroadenomas do not show any vascularity around or within them on Doppler studies (Plate C.8.a), but occasionally feeding vessels can be seen in young subjects and in large lesions (Plate C.8.b).

The reported incidence of ultrasound features of fibroadenomas is listed in Table 5.1.

Fig. 5.10
Compressibility and mobility of a fibroadenoma
This fibroadenoma with typical appearances (**a**) deforms and revolves when a twisting movement is applied by the free hand (**b**).

Fa: fibroadenoma.

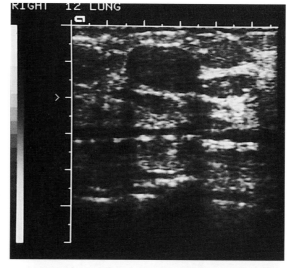
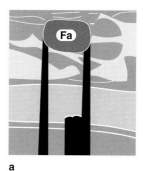

a

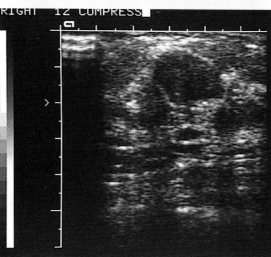
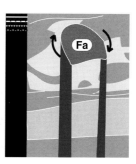

b

Fig. 5.11
Compressibility of a fibroadenoma
This oval fibroadenoma (**a**) deforms when compressed from the sides (**b**), indicating a soft consistency. Such compressibility is rarely seen in carcinomas.

Fa: fibroadenoma
Gl: mammary gland

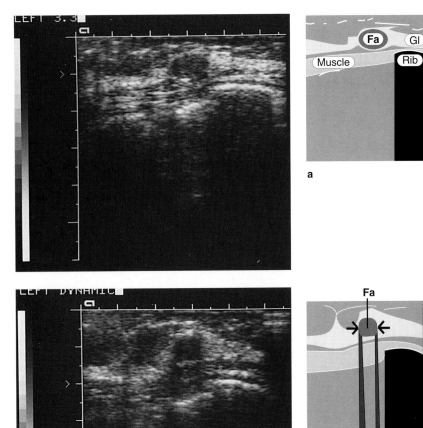

a

b

Table 5.1	Ultrasound features of fibroadenomas			
	Cole-Beuglet[6] N=140	**Heywang[7]** N=30	**Jackson[3]** N=76	**Fornage[4]** N=101
Undetected	18%	20%	18%	1%
Shape				
Round	48%	75%	47%	57%*
Oval	37%	–	–	–
Lobulated	15%	–	31%	16%
Internal echoes				
Echo-poor	80%	96%	–	92%
Isoechoic (= fat)	11%	–	–	1%
Echogenic	–	–	–	4%
Texture				
Uniform	88%	75%	48%	71%
Edge				
Smooth	75%	63%	42%	–
Edge shadows	–	50%	–	–
Posterior echoes				
Enhancement	20%	33%	24%	17%
Intermediate	71%	29%	–	73%
Shadowing	9%	–	11%	10%

* Interpreted as a regular shape.

Giant fibroadenoma

Occasionally fibroadenomas reach a considerable size, though size alone is not an indicator of malignancy. There is no agreed definition for the term 'giant fibroadenoma' which has sometimes been applied to phylloides tumours as well as to otherwise ordinary fibroadenomas 6 cm or more in diameter[8].

Histologically giant fibroadenomas are simply large fibroadenomas. The ultrasound appearances are also the same as those of common fibroadenoma except for their large size[9] (Fig. 5.12). Some are highly vascular.

Juvenile fibroadenoma

Not all fibroadenomas found in adolescents belong in this category, most being of the adult type. Juvenile fibroadenomas grow rapidly and may arouse suspicion of malignancy on clinical examination, although the rarity of breast carcinomas or phylloides tumours in this age group is reassuring.

Histologically this term is used to describe tumours of high cellularity in adolescents (Plate P.5.2). Care should be taken to distinguish lesions with densely cellular stroma from phylloides tumours, especially in older patients.

Fig. 5.12
Giant fibroadenomas
Fibroadenomas larger than 6 cm in diameter are often called 'giant' (**a**, **b**). Apart from their large size, the appearances are typical of a fibroadenoma (oval shape with homogeneous echoes). Increased vascularity may be seen in tumours of this size.

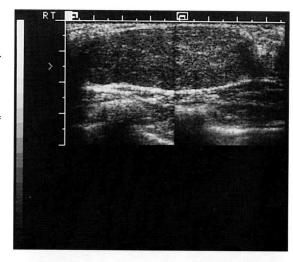
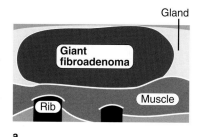

a

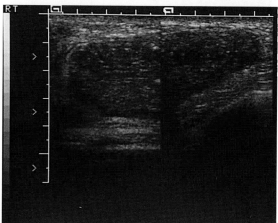
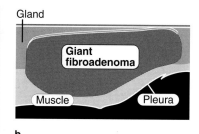

b

On ultrasound, they are usually of moderate to large size but otherwise have the same general appearances as ordinary fibroadenomas. However, they have a deeper AP diameter and almost always show strong posterior enhancement. A striking finding is their increased vascularity on Doppler studies, probably corresponding to their rapid growth (Plate C.8).

Lactating fibroadenoma
Fibroadenomas may grow rapidly in the first half of preg-

nancy. Histologically the epithelial elements undergo secretory changes and produce milk proteins. Extension of the epithelial tissue into the surrounding fat and marked mitotic activity may raise the suspicion of malignancy.

On ultrasound they cannot be differentiated from giant or juvenile fibroadenomas or even from phylloides tumours (Fig. 5.13).

Fig. 5.13
Lactating fibroadenoma
In the third month of her pregnancy this lady noticed a breast lump which gradually enlarged. As with juvenile fibroadenomas, they often grow rapidly and may reach a considerable size. Histologically marked pleomorphism may suggest the possibility of a low grade phylloides tumour but this patient had no signs of recurrence after excision biopsy.

PE: posterior enhancement

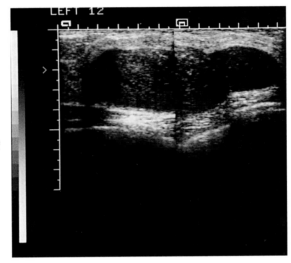
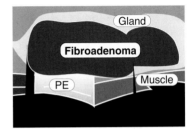

REFERENCES

1. C.D. Haagensen: Diseases of the Breast (3rd edn). W.B. Saunders, Philadelphia, 1986, pp 267–283.
2. K. Buzanowski-Kanakry, E.G. Harrison, W.S. Payne: Lobular carcinoma arising in fibroadenoma of the breast. Cancer 35; 450–456, 1975.
3. V.P. Jackson, P.A. Rothschild, D.L. Kreipke, et al: The spectrum of sonographic findings of fibroadenoma of the breast. Invest Radiol 21; 34–40, 1986.
4. B.D. Fornage, J.G. Lorigan, E. Andry: Fibroadenoma of the breast: sonographic appearance. Radiology 172; 671–675, 1989.
5. B.J. Hackelöer, V. Duda, G. Lauth: Ultrasound Mammography. Springer-Verlag, Berlin, 1986, pp 34–40.
6. C. Cole-Beuglet, R.Z. Soriano, A.B. Kurtz, B.B. Goldberg: Fibroadenoma of the breast: sonomammography correlated with pathology in 122 patients. AJR 140; 369–375, 1983.
7. S.H. Heywang, E.R. Lipsit, L.M. Glassman, M.T. Thomas: Specificity of ultrasonography in the diagnosis of benign breast masses. J Ultrasound Med 3; 453–461, 1984.
8. C.S. Moran: Fibroadenoma of the breast during pregnancy and lactation. Arch Surg 31; 688–708, 1935.
9. R.T. Steinbock, P.C. Stomper, J.E. Meyer, D.B. Kopans: The ultrasound appearance of giant fibroadenoma. J Clin Ultrasound 11; 451–454, 1983.

5.2 PHYLLOIDES TUMOUR

CLINICAL FEATURES

Phylloides tumour, also known as 'cystosarcoma phylloides', is uncommon. It resembles a fibroadenoma both clinically and pathologically and has been called 'giant fibroadenoma' by some workers — an unsuitable term as phylloides tumours may be small and fibroadenomas large, particularly in juveniles.

Phylloides tumours may occur at any age, the median being about 45 years, which is significantly higher than that for fibroadenomas. Presentation is almost always with a lump of variable but often large size. On palpation, the lesion is well-circumscribed and not adherent to the chest wall or skin. Very large tumours may occasionally cause ulceration of the skin by extreme stretching rather than by invasion. Bilateral or multiple lesions are rare. About 20% of these tumours behave in a malignant fashion[10], tending to recur locally or to spread haematogenously, mainly to lung, pleura and bone; axillary lymph node metastases are rare.

PATHOLOGICAL FEATURES

Phylloides tumours are composed of epithelial and stromal elements and have the same basic structure as intracanalicular fibroadenomas. They appear well-circumscribed on macroscopic examination but at microscopic level there are often irregular rounded projections from the surface, or truly infiltrative margins. A characteristic feature of many tumours is the presence of leaf-like processes projecting into cystic spaces, from which the tumour derives its name (Plate P.5.3).

The essential point of distinction from fibroadenoma is the greater cellularity of the stroma which varies considerably from tumour to tumour and even within the same lesion. Low and high grade variants are recognised. In the former, the stroma has the appearance of a cellular fibroma and lacks cytological evidence of malignancy. In the latter, it resembles a sarcoma (Plate P.5.4). Although the stroma usually has a non-specific spindle cell appearance,

differentiation towards fat, smooth muscle, cartilage and bone have been reported[11]. The epithelium is usually similar to that in the normal breast although there may be zones of hyperplasia which are occasionally atypical. There are cases on record of carcinoma developing within a phylloides tumour, but they are rare[11].

Separating these tumours into high and low grade variants on histological grounds has been disappointingly ineffective in predicting outcome. Recurrence and metastasis have been observed in both groups[11,12]. Where histological features have been studied in detail, however, small size, low mitotic rate, 'pushing' rather than infiltrative margins and minimal cytological atypia have been found to be associated with low risk of recurrence but no feature is wholly reliable and a clear-cut separation into benign and malignant cannot be made on histology.

ULTRASOUND FEATURES

The morphological appearances are almost identical to those of fibroadenomas[13] (Fig. 5.14). They tend to be large masses with an oval, round or lobulated shape. They are well-circumscribed and do not have a halo. There is usually posterior enhancement. Some authors have described the presence of slit-like fluid-filled spaces[14,15]; when seen they are diagnostic, but the internal echoes are usually homogeneous. In large tumours, necrosis or haemorrhage make the internal echoes heterogeneous but calcifications are not seen, nor are secondary features of invasion.

Increased vascularity has been observed in and around phylloides tumours on colour Doppler (Plate C.10). This is not a specific feature because large fibroadenomas may also have increased vascularity, but it may represent proliferative activity and the possibility of a phylloides tumour must be considered when marked vascularity is found in a fibroadenoma-like tumour, especially in a middle-aged woman.

REFERENCES

10. H.J. Norris, H.B. Taylor: Relationship of histologic features to behaviour of cystosarcoma phylloides: analysis of ninety-four cases. Cancer 20; 2090–2099, 1967
11. K.D.L. Lindquist, J.A. van Heerden, J.H. Weiland, J.K. Martin: Recurrent and metastatic cystosarcoma phylloides. Am J Surg 144; 341–343, 1982.
12. S.I. Hajdu, M.H. Espinosa, G.F. Robbins: Recurrent cystosarcoma phylloides: a clinicopathologic study of 32 cases. Cancer 38: 1402–1406, 1976.

13. C. Cole-Beuglet, R. Soriano, A.B. Kurtz et al: Ultrasound, X-ray mammography, and histopathology of cystosarcoma phylloides. Radiology 146; 481–486, 1983
14. D.B. Kopans: Breast Imaging. J.B. Lippincott, Philadelphia, 1989.
15. F. Kasumi: Ultrasound of the Breast Lesions. Shinohara-shuppan, Tokyo, 1983.

Fig. 5.14
Phylloides tumours

a. This 4.5 cm × 2 cm tumour has an oval shape with homogeneous internal echoes and posterior enhancement. These appearances are identical of those of a large fibroadenoma but a new mass in a 38-year-old woman warrants removal. Histologically this was a high grade phylloides tumour.

b. Small phylloides tumour. This lesion was not seen on an ultrasound examination a year before but its appearances are also those of a benign lesion. Because cytology of this was C4, it was removed and on histology a low grade phylloides tumour was found.

c. Lobulated phylloides tumour. This lesion is lobular but not irregular in shape. It has slightly heterogeneous internal texture with posterior enhancement. These appearances are consistent with a phylloides tumour or a fibroadenoma; the former was suggested because of the patient's age (58 years). Histologically this was a high grade phylloides tumour.

ES: edge shadow
GI: mammary gland
SCF: subcutaneous fat

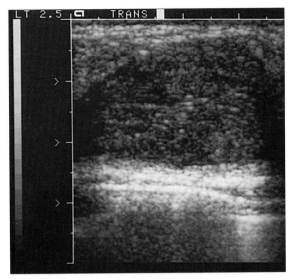
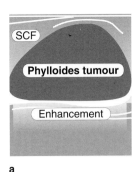

a

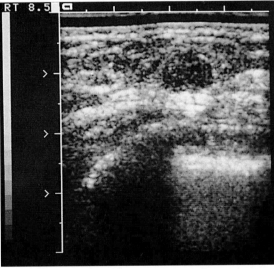
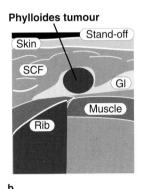

b

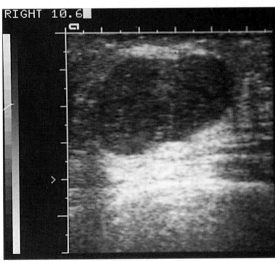
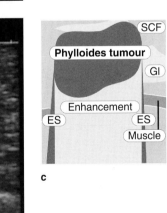

c

5.3 INTRADUCT PAPILLOMA

CLINICAL FEATURES

Intraduct papillomas are relatively common with a reported incidence of one to ten carcinomas[16], though they are more common as incidental findings in biopsy specimens, particularly in the elderly[17]. Though benign, they cause problems because of their similarity to intraduct papillary carcinoma clinically, ultrasonographically and even histologically. They may occur at any age but are most common between 35 and 55 years.

The characteristic clinical features are nipple discharge and a tumour mass; these coexist in 30%, with discharge alone and tumour alone accounting for 40% and 30% of cases respectively[16]. The discharge may be serous or blood-stained. Most intraduct papillomas develop under the nipple or in the subareolar region because they arise from the larger lactiferous ducts. One useful method to localise the site of a non-palpable lesion is to locate a 'trigger point' along the areolar border that results in expression of fluid from the nipple.

PATHOLOGICAL FEATURES

On macroscopic examination, a papilloma may appear as an elongated structure (usually a few millimetres in diameter) extending along the duct system or as a larger and more spheroidal lesion. The latter type results in greater distension of the duct which, in some cases, assumes a cyst-like appearance. The term 'intracystic papilloma' is often used to describe this variant (Plate P.5.5). Histologically papillomas have an arborescent growth pattern with branching fibrovascular cores of myoepithelial and epithelial cells. The cytological features are benign but necrosis and haemorrhage are not infrequent and may lead to fibrosis. Irregular zones of fibrosis around the periphery may obscure the margin of the tumour and give a false impression of invasion. Chondroid and osseous metaplasia may rarely occur[18].

ULTRASOUND FEATURES

Three patterns are recognised on ultrasonography: intraductal, intracystic and solid[19] (Fig. 5.15). Pneumocystography, previously considered the 'gold standard' for this lesion, has been replaced by ultrasound which is simpler and equally sensitive in the diagnosis of intraduct tumours[20–22]. It is important that the ultrasound be performed before cyst puncture, since the bleeding caused by needling may obscure the cystic component around the papilloma, or may produce an apparent soft tissue mass within a simple cyst.

Previously, ultrasound was considered to be less useful in cases without a palpable mass and, although some lesions are difficult to detect, dilated ducts can easily be detected and traced with high resolution real-time equipment so that impalpable tumours can now be identified. An important practical point is to avoid squeezing the duct (e.g. to obtain a cytological specimen) before the ultrasound examination, since the empty ducts are almost

impossible to visualise and the associated abnormalities disappear completely. The transducer must touch the skin very lightly during scanning and extra gel used in order not to compress the ducts.

If the tumour itself is very small, only dilated ducts are seen. This should not be mistaken for major duct ectasia, a chronic inflammatory condition in which the collecting ducts and lactiferous sinuses are filled with creamy secretions, in which multiple ducts are affected bilaterally (see Ch. 7). A single dilated duct in a patient with nipple discharge is a suspicious combination, particularly if the discharge is blood-stained. Ductal carcinoma in situ may also produce dilated ducts filled with tumour which, in the comedo variant, exhibits central necrosis. Duct dilatation tends to be more extensive and irregular in carcinomas and is usually more peripheral.

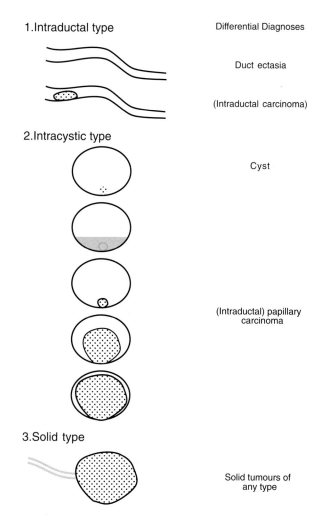

Fig. 5.15
Ultrasonic appearances of intraduct papilloma

Dilated ducts with a solid component are typical of an intraductal papilloma (Fig. 5.16) and, if associated with nipple discharge, biopsy is required. In major duct ectasia, branching, tortuousity or focal dilatation may produce apparent intraductal soft tissue masses. In these cases the solid parts are not real but are caused by the scan plane passing through the edge of the tortuous duct wall. Careful tracing along the duct should solve this problem. Inspissated material in ectatic ducts may have a similar appearance but the echogenic portions are not as distinct as in true solid lesions.

The 'cysts' in the intracystic type are actually formed by focally dilated ducts. Solid masses within cysts are typ-

ical of intraductal papillomas (Fig. 5.17). The masses may be very small (in which case it is easily missed, the lesion being mistaken for a simple cyst) or be large enough to occupy almost the entire cavity. The distinction from intracystic papillary carcinoma usually cannot be made on ultrasound, though the older age distribution of the malignant type is a useful guide (see section on 'nipple discharge'). A fluid–fluid level, which represents bleeding into the cyst, is a feature that should arouse a strong suspicion of a mural proliferative lesion; most commonly this will be an intraductal papillary carcinoma but it can also be found with a papilloma.

Fig. 5.16
Intraduct papilloma (intraduct type)
This patient presented with bloody nipple discharge. No mass was palpable. A solid tumour is seen in a dilated duct in the subareolar region. On histology an intraduct papilloma was found.

IDP: intraduct papilloma

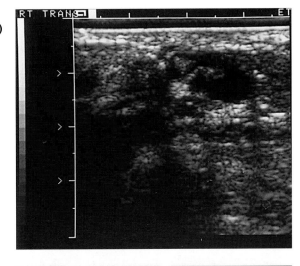
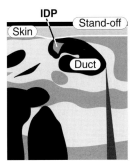

Fig. 5.17
Intraduct papilloma (intracystic type)
This subareolar mass has both solid and cystic components. The appearance and site are typical of an intraduct papilloma.

ES: edge shadow
IDP: intraduct papilloma
PE: posterior enhancement
RMS: retromammary space

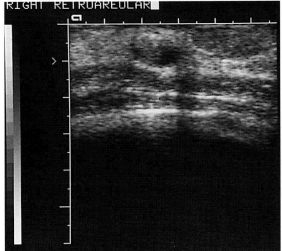
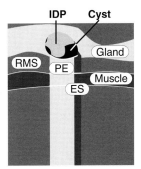

An intraductal papilloma may be visualised as a solid tumour. They are usually small (<2 cm), located close to the nipple and produce distal enhancement. The appearances are non-specific but demonstration of a dilated duct nearby increases the likelihood of finding an intraductal papilloma (Fig. 5.18).

MULTIPLE INTRADUCT PAPILLOMA

Multiple intraduct papilloma is a rare entity in which many adjacent ducts are involved and the changes extend away from the nipple. The incidence of nipple discharge is lower than with intraductal papillomas (30–50%)[16,23]. Palpable masses are often found in the peripheral portions of the breast. Histologically, the lesions are identical to ordinary papillomas. The problem with this lesion is the high risk of associated malignancy, the incidence being reported as about 30%[16,23]. No special ultrasound appearances have been noted.

JUVENILE PAPILLOMATOSIS

Juvenile papillomatosis is a rare condition also known as 'Swiss cheese disease' because of its characteristic pathological appearances. Despite its name, there is a wide age distribution from about 10 to 48 years though 70% of patients are under 26 years[24,25]. It usually presents as a peripherally located palpable mass resembling a fibroadenoma. A quarter of patients have a family history of breast carcinomas and about 4% also have carcinoma at presentation, sometimes in the contralateral breast[25].

Pathologically, juvenile papillomatosis is characterised by cysts, duct ectasia, intraductal hyperplasia and sclerosing adenosis (Plate P.5.6). Although none of these changes is specific for the condition, the combination of features and the age at presentation make it a distinctive disorder. The large number of cysts and dilated ducts produce the characteristic appearance of Swiss cheese.

One report about ultrasound features describes an ill-defined heterogeneous mass associated with several small, rounded, relatively echo-free areas near the margins[26].

NIPPLE DISCHARGE

Not all nipple discharge is pathological. For example newborn babies may secrete milk under the influence of maternal hormones ('witch's milk'), and during pregnancy a nipple discharge, sometimes bloody, may occur. Even in non-lactating, non-pregnant women, fluid secretion from the nipple is not uncommon, and by using a special suction device Love et al obtained specimens in 83% of unselected non-pregnant women[24]. Habitual squeezing also induces nipple discharge so that only spontaneous nipple discharge is clinically significant.

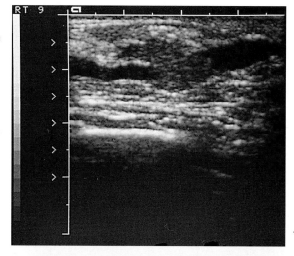
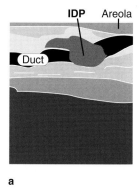
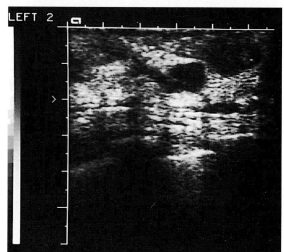
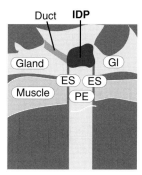

Fig. 5.18
Intraduct papilloma (solid type)
a. A tumour close to the nipple is seen to be originating from the duct. Because the solid portion is larger than the duct (the tumour seems to invade the adjacent stroma), a papillary carcinoma was suspected but on histology it proved to be an intraduct papilloma. The differentiation between papilloma and papillary carcinoma is very difficult on ultrasound.
b. A dilated duct lies between this echo-poor mass and the nipple, suggesting the diagnosis of an intraduct papilloma despite the lack of a cystic component. Note the distal enhancement.

ES: edge shadow
GI: mammary gland
IDP: intraduct papilloma
PE: posterior enhancement

Bilateral milky discharge from multiple ducts other than during pregnancy and lactation (galactorrhoea) is usually endocrine induced, often associated with hyperprolactin-aemia though pituitary adenomas account for only 2% of all cases of galactorrhoea[28]. Many drugs are known to cause hyperprolactinaemia and thereby galactorrhoea; examples include psychotropic agents (major tranquillis-ers), antihypertensives and oral contraceptives.

Nipple discharge due to breast pathology characteristi-cally occurs from a single duct. Patients who have a pal-pable mass associated with a discharge do not pose spe-cial diagnostic problems because the mass requires evalu-ation in its own right. Nipple discharge without a palpa-ble mass remains a diagnostic challenge. The discharge may be bloody (including serosanguineous) or serous. A test for occult blood may be used to differentiate between them[29].

The commonest causes for nipple discharge are intra-ductal papillomas and carcinomas (many are of the in situ type). Intraductal papilloma accounts for more than 50% and carcinomas are found in some 20%, the incidence increasing with age and when the discharge is bloody[29–32]. Bloody discharge occurs because of haemorrhagic necro-sis of a part of a papilloma or carcinoma. Benign breast change may also produce nipple discharge, especially when associated with duct ectasia; the fluid is typically turbid and yellow, green, brown or black in colour.

Cytology of the fluid is disappointing because degener-ation of the cells makes differentiation between benign and malignant difficult; canulating the duct and aspirat-ing the fluid directly provides slightly better specimens, but the sensitivity remains low at 20–40%[33,34]. Assay of carcinoembryonic antigen in the discharge has also been used but is not very helpful. Ductography can demon-strate intraduct lesions and duct distortion but the proce-dure itself may cause an inflammatory reaction. Micro-dochectomy or tumour excision is appropriate treatment that also provides the diagnosis. Microdochectomy is per-formed by inserting a blunt needle or lacrimal probe into the discharging duct which is then dissected and excised, together with a cone of underlying breast tissue.

There are few reports on the ultrasound appearances or its usefulness in the diagnosis of nipple discharge[35,36]. The ultrasound features are summarised in Table 5.2.

Table 5.2 Ultrasonic features in nipple discharge

Findings	Cause
Dilated duct only	Single—Non-specific, but possibility of intraductal proliferative lesion Multiple—Benign breast change (duct ectasia)
Dilated duct with intraductal or intracystic masses	Papillary tumours, including intraductal papilloma, multiple papillomas, papillary carcinoma
Dilated duct and mass Mass	Papillary tumours and invasive carcinoma with ductal spread

REFERENCES

16. C.D. Haagensen: Diseases of the Breast (3rd edn). W.B. Saunders, Philadelphia, 1986, pp 136–175.
17. W.M. Kramer, B.F. Rush: Mammary duct proliferation in the elderly: a histopathologic study. Cancer 31; 130–137, 1973.
18. B.H. Smith, H.B. Taylor: The occurrence of bone and cartilage in mammary tumors. Am J Clin Pathol 51; 610–618, 1969.
19. F. Kasumi: Ultrasound of Breast Diseases. Shinohara-shuppan Co., Tokyo, 1983.
20. L. Tabár, Z. Péntek, P.B. Dean: The diagnostic and therapeutic value of breast cyst puncture and pneumocystography. Radiology 141; 659–663, 1981.
21. U. Dyreborg, M. Blichert-Toft, L. Boegh, H. Kiaer: Needle puncture followed by pneumocystography of palpable breast cysts: a controlled clinical trial. Acta Radiol Diag 26; 277–281, 1985.
22. K. Reuter, C.J. D'Orsi, F. Reale: Intracystic carcinoma of the breast: the role of ultrasonography. Radiology 153; 233–234, 1984.
23. T.M. Murad, G. Contesso, H. Mouriesse: Papillary tumors of large lactiferous ducts. Cancer 48; 122–133, 1981.
24. P.P. Rosen, B. Cantrell, D.L. Mullen, A. DePalo: Juvenile papillo-matosis (Swiss cheese disease) of the breast. Am J Surg Pathol 4; 3–12, 1980.
25. P.P. Rosen, G. Holmes, M.L. Lesser, et al: Juvenile papillomatosis and breast carcinoma. Cancer 55; 1345–1352, 1985.
26. E.A.J. Kersschot, M. Hermans, C. Pauwels, et al: Juvenile papillo-matosis of the breast: sonographic appearance. Radiology 169; 631–633, 1988.
27. S.M. Love, S.J. Schnitt, J.L. Connolly, R.L. Shirley: Benign breast disorders. In: Breast Diseases, edited by J.R. Harris, S. Hellman, I.C. Henderson, D.W. Kinne. J.B. Lippincott, Philadelphia, 1987, pp 15–53.
28. Editorial: Discharge from the nipple. Lancet ii; 1405, 1983.
29. M.A. Chaudary, R.R. Millis, G.C. Davies, J.L. Hayward: Nipple discharge: the diagnostic value of testing for occult blood. Ann Surg 196; 651–655, 1982.
30. C.D. Haagensen: Diseases of the Breast (3rd edn). W.B. Saunders, Philadelphia, 1986, pp 503–504.
31. A.P. Locker, M.H. Galea, I.O. Ellis, et al: Microdochectomy for single-duct discharge from the nipple. Br J Surg 75; 700–701, 1988.
32. M.H. Seltzer, L.J. Perloff, R.I. Kelley, W.T. Fitts: The significance of age in patients with nipple discharge. Surg Gynecol Obstet 140; 519–522, 1970.
33. E.B. King, K.L. Chew, N.L. Petrakis, V.L. Ernster: Nipple aspirate cytology for the study of breast cancer precursors. JNCI 71; 1115–1121, 1983.
34. E.B. King, D. Barrett, N.L. Petrakis: Cellular composition of the nipple aspirate specimen of breast fluid: II. Abnormal findings. AJCP 64; 739–748, 1975.
35. H.S. Tsunoda, E. Ueno, E. Tohno, et al: Clinical significance of demonstration of the dilated duct on real time echogram in cases of abnormal nipple discharge. Jpn J Med Ultrasonics 16 (suppl I); 295–296, 1989.
36. T. Kamio, S. Kameoka, H. Kanzaki, et al: Ultrasonographic diagnosis of nonpalpable breast tumors in patients with abnormal nipple discharge. Jpn J Med Ultrasonics 16; 463–470, 1989.

5.4 LIPOMA AND FIBROADENOLIPOMA

LIPOMA

CLINICAL FEATURES

Lipomas are common benign mesenchymal (non-epithelial) neoplasms, found in any part of the body where fat occurs and particularly commonly on the shoulders or back. Lipomas in the breast are difficult to distinguish from redundant fatty tissue, unless they are large. Most develop in the subcutaneous fat but they are occasionally encountered within the gland itself or deep to the muscular fascia.

They present as superficially located, soft and lobulated mobile masses which do not produce dimpling or nipple retraction. Because they are not glandular in origin, lipomas often occur in the periphery of the breast, on the chest wall or in the axillary region.

On mammograms lipomas have the same radiolucency as surrounding fatty tissue but can be distinguished from normal fatty tissues by a delicate capsule (Fig. 5.19).

PATHOLOGICAL FEATURES

The majority of lipomas consist almost entirely of mature adipocytes indistinguishable from those seen in normal adipose tissue. Consequently, it may be difficult or impossible to distinguish lipomas from normal fat on histological grounds except that they are usually encapsulated and rather more vascular than normal adipose tissue.

Several uncommon variants have been described: (1) angiolipomas in which a network of small blood vessels is prominent, (2) spindle cell lipoma which consists of variable proportions of collagen-forming spindle cells and mature adipocytes, and (3) pleomorphic lipoma consisting of mixtures of adipocytes, spindle cells and distinctive multinucleate giant cells. Variants 2 and 3, however, usually occur in the neck and shoulder region of males, rather than in the breast.

Fig. 5.19
Lipoma within the glandular layer
A lipoma has the same radiolucency
as the fatty tissue but is recognisable
mammographically because of its thin
capsule, especially when it lies in the
glandular layer of the breast (**a**).
Intraglandular lipomas are difficult to
distinguish from the normal fatty
tissue or fibroadenomas on
ultrasound; this lesion was only
detected after comparison with the
mammogram. The lipoma is seen as
a lens-shaped, homogeneous
structure with an echogenicity slightly
higher than that of the surrounding
fatty tissue (**b**).

Gl: mammary gland
SCF: subcutaneous fat

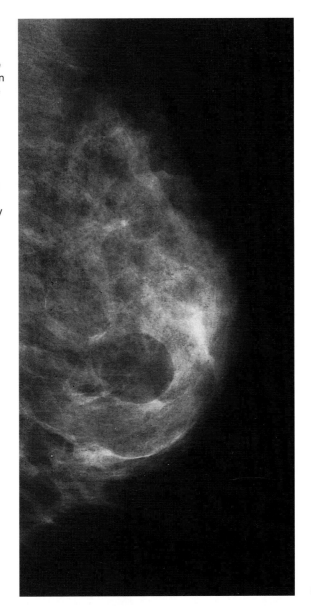

a

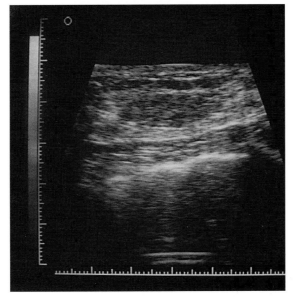

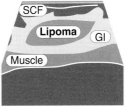

b

ULTRASOUND FEATURES

Lipomas may be found in any of the layers of the breast (anterior to the superficial layer of the superficial fascia, between its two layers or deep to the deep layer), in contrast to disorders of the specialised mammary stroma and epithelium which always originate between the two layers. They are usually oval or lenticular in shape and well-circumscribed. As expected, lipomas usually return the same echo levels as fat but, for unknown reasons, echogenic and echo-poor variants are encountered. The internal texture is homogeneous and there are no secondary features because the mass does not elicit a reaction from the surrounding tissue. Lipomas are easily compressible since the fat they contain is actually an oil at body temperature.

Homogeneous echogenic masses in the subcutaneous fatty tissue layer are relatively easy to recognise and, if they do not have posterior attenuation, the appearance is almost specific for a lipoma (Fig. 5.20). Other breast masses are usually echo-poor, except for granulomas and calcific breast carcinomas both of which produce strong posterior attenuation. Fibroadenomas are occasionally echogenic, but this variety is very rare. Lipomas of the same echogenicity as the surrounding fatty tissue are very difficult to recognise, especially in involuted breasts, unless they are large enough to displace the normal structures or can be located by palpation in which case they are obvious clinically (Fig. 5.21). Small lipomas are probably often missed on ultrasound, being interpreted as normal fatty tissue. Echo-poor lipomas are almost identical to fibroadenomas in appearance though their marked compressibility may indicate their true nature; mammograms are useful to confirm the diagnosis because fibroadenomas have soft tissue density while lipomas are radiolucent. Ultrasound may detect asymptomatic lipomas, but they are clinically not important.

FIBROADENOLIPOMA

CLINICAL AND PATHOLOGICAL FEATURES

Fibroadenolipomas are a rare type of fatty tumour, peculiar to the breast. They consist of a mixture of fat and epithelial elements together with fibrous tissue. They may be called adenolipomas if the fibrous component is lacking (Plate P.5.7)[37,38]. It is unlikely that all the components are neoplastic, the glandular and fibrous elements probably simply being incorporated into a fatty tumour.

The mammographic features are pathognomonic: they are seen as well-delimited masses composed of dysplastic-appearing mammary tissue admixed with fat[39]. In typical cases surgical removal is not necessary, although the mammographic appearances are not always classical[40].

The term 'hamartoma' is used to describe a clinically discrete nodule of very variable size, consisting of normal breast lobules surrounded by normal fibroadipose stroma. The lesion thus appears to represent a local overgrowth of histologically normal breast tissue. Although sharply delineated, hamartomas do not usually have a fibrous capsule.

ULTRASOUND FEATURES

Few reports are available on the ultrasonographic features of fibroadenolipoma. A wide spectrum of ultrasonographic appearances has been reported, the most frequent being a moderate to well-circumscribed solid, echo-poor mass with posterior shadowing[41,42]. The range of the appearances is presumably due to variations in the proportions of the constituent elements; the fact that lipomas, (fibro)adenolipomas and hamartomas are confused in the literature probably also accounts for some of the variability. The differentiation between fat and epithelial or fibrotic tissue is not as reliable on ultrasound as on mammography.

REFERENCES

37. J.E. Spalding: Adeno-lipoma and lipoma of the breast. Guy's Hosp Rep 94; 80–84, 1945.
38. M.G. Arrigoni, M.B. Dockerty, E.S. Judd: The identification and treatment of mammary hamartoma. Surg Gynecol and Obstet 133; 577–582, 1971.
39. C. Hessler, P. Schnyder, L. Ozzello: Hamartoma of the breast: diagnostic observation of 16 cases. Radiology 126; 95–98, 1978.
40. M.A. Helvie, D.D. Adler, M. Rebner, H.A. Oberman: Breast hamartomas: variable mammographic appearances. Radiology 170; 417–421, 1989.
41. D.B. Kopans, J.E. Meyer, K.H. Proppe: Ultrasonographic, xeromammographic and histologic correlation of a fibroadenolipoma of the breast. J Clin Ultrasound 10; 409–411, 1982.
42. D.D. Adler, D.O. Jeffries, M.A. Helvie: Sonographic features of breast hamartomas. J Ultrasound Med 9; 85–90, 1990.

Fig. 5.20
Echogenic lipomas in the subcutaneous fat
Echogenic lipomas are easily detected (**a**, **b**). Echogenic lesions of the breast are rare and the anterior location of these masses would be unusual for tumours of the gland itself. This appearance is almost specific for a lipoma.

SCF: subcutaneous fat
SL: superficial layer of the superficial fascia
RMS: retromammary space

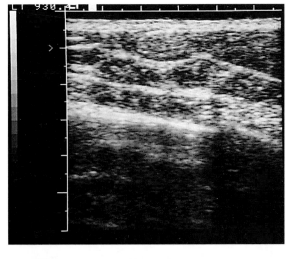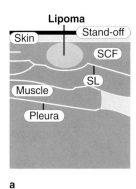

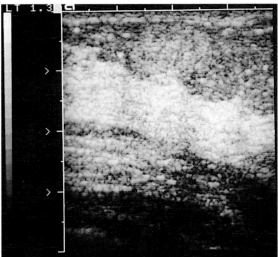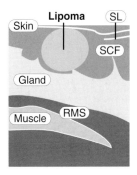

Fig. 5.21
Isoechoic lipoma
A large, soft mass in the medial part of the breast was considered clinically to be a lipoma. On ultrasound the mass has almost the same appearance as a normal fatty lobule but is larger and more homogeneous in texture, presumably because it lacks the fibrous components of normal adipose tissue.

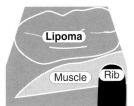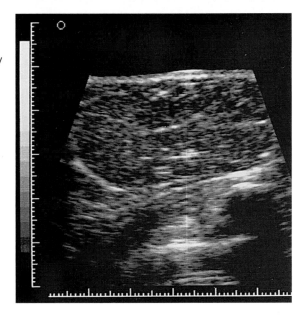

Chapter 6

Benign processes – cysts, benign breast change, gynaecomastia

6.1 CYSTS

CLINICAL FEATURES

Although cysts are one component of benign breast change which is described later in this chapter, they have particular features both clinically and ultrasonographically and are therefore described separately. Cysts are perhaps the commonest cause of a breast lump and need to be distinguished from more important masses such as fibroadenomas and particularly carcinomas.

Cysts and fibroadenomas most commonly occur in the 35–55 age group, whereas carcinomas predominate in older women (over the age of 50). Cysts usually do not increase in size or number after the menopause, an exception being their occasional appearance de novo in women receiving hormone replacement therapy. There is still much uncertainty about the detailed mechanisms of cyst production — physiological changes are probably partly responsible.

Cysts are usually asymptomatic and are found incidentally (e.g. on palpation) but may cause pain if leakage or rupture occurs or when they are very tense. Cysts may appear in a few days or even overnight, the sudden onset distinguishing them from neoplasms.

On palpation cysts are usually round, smooth and well-circumscribed. Their consistency is variable, mainly depending on their internal pressure; tense cysts are as firm as a carcinoma. When lax, they are soft and often completely impalpable. Fluctuation, one of the most characteristic features of cysts, is demonstrated on bimanual palpation, compressing the cyst with the finger of one hand. Cysts are usually attached to the surrounding breast tissue at least to some extent and so are not as mobile as fibroadenomas.

The contents of cysts have a wide range of appearances from clear to turbid, from straw-coloured through brown to almost black. If the fluid is blood-stained, cytological examination should be performed to exclude an intracystic tumour, but cysts with clear fluid are always simple so that cytology is unnecessary.

PATHOLOGICAL FEATURES

Cysts are extremely common histological findings and increase in incidence with age up to the menopause. However, only a few attain a sufficient size and tension to be clinically detectable. They arise by dilatation and co-alescence of the acini of terminal duct lobular units (TDLUs); thus, they are often found in clusters although they may be solitary, especially if expansion is marked. Small cysts may occur as part of breast involution but larger ones are generally thought to arise as a proliferative process. Obstruction of ducts by epithelial hyperplasia or stromal fibrosis are not now considered to be important in the pathogenesis of cysts. The possible role of ducts cannot be completely discounted as secretion by TDLUs and reabsorption and drainage by ducts are balanced in the normal situation and blockage of outflow may contribute to cyst formation.

Their epithelial lining frequently shows metaplasia to cells resembling those of normal apocrine sweat glands with large rounded nuclei and copious granular eosinophilic cytoplasm. These cells usually form a single layer but papillary tufting may be seen (Plate P.6.1). As cysts enlarge, the epithelium may become attenuated or even disappear. Such cysts usually contain fluid under pressure and are known as 'tension cysts'. The walls of cysts are usually devoid of fibrosis, elastosis or inflammation unless leakage of cyst contents has taken place.

ULTRASONIC FEATURES

Cysts are very common findings on breast ultrasound. In a series of 300 studies, one-quarter of all palpable masses and non-palpable, mammographically dominant masses were confirmed to be cysts on ultrasound[1]. On the other hand, not all apparently cystic nodularity of the breast is actually due to cysts; heterogeneous consistency of the glandular tissue sometimes simulates cysts on palpation. Cysts lying deep in the glandular tissue may be misinterpreted as solid masses, especially when fluid cannot be aspirated. Superimposed glandular tissues may be misinterpreted as nodular densities that suggest cysts on mammograms.

Cysts are also commonly found on ultrasound in asymptomatic women. When one or a few cysts are palpable, the mammogram may show several cysts, but usually many more cysts are demonstrated on ultrasound. Cysts have been reported in 20% of asymptomatic women with dense breasts on mammography[2]. In homogeneously echogenic glandular tissue, cysts as small as 2 mm in diameter can easily be recognised with high resolution scanners. It has been said that cysts are rare in young women; however, on ultrasound they are not infrequently encountered in women in their twenties.

Ultrasound is highly reliable in the diagnosis of cysts, the accuracy being reported as 98–100%[3,4]. Cysts with typical appearances are readily diagnosed with high specificity. This type is called a 'simple cyst' and does not need biopsy or further investigation since there is negligible risk of confusion with significant pathology. However, ultrasound is less specific for cysts with atypical appearances, whether due to real abnormalities or to artefacts,

Table 6.1	Differential diagnosis of 'cysts' (pathologies which mimic cysts or contain cystic areas)
Intracystic tumours, e.g. intraductal papilloma or papillary carcinoma	
Necrotic tumours	
Abscess	
Haematoma, postsurgical or posttraumatic	
Fat necrosis (oil cyst)	
Prosthesis	
Cellular tumours, e.g. lymphoma, medullary carcinoma	

so that needle aspiration is required, though there may be clues that may allow a differentiation from malignant lesions.

Other pathologies which must be distinguished from cysts are listed in Table 6.1. The ultrasound features of these diseases are described in their respective sections.

SIMPLE CYSTS

Because absence of reflections is one of the conspicuous characteristics of fluid, the echo-free nature of the contents of the lesion is the most important diagnostic feature. However, there are several additional features, which are helpful in the differentiation of cysts from other pathologies. The typical appearances of cysts (Fig. 6.1) are:

1. Echo-free contents
2. Posterior enhancement
3. Smooth, thin walls
4. Edge shadows

Cysts are virtually the only structures that are truly anechoic. The only exceptions are the rare purely cellular tumours without stroma, such as malignant lymphoma or medullary carcinoma, which may have extremely low internal echoes that may be difficult to distinguish from noise. They may also show posterior enhancement which adds to the difficulty. However, they usually have a more irregular shape than cysts, are incompressible and may show blood flow within the 'echo-free' area on Doppler, all of which help avoid misinterpretation. Breast carcinomas with strong attenuation may often seem to be echo-free but here the cause is completely different, being due to strong shadowing. Because the main part of the mass is 'self shadowed' by its strongly attenuating anterior part, distal shadowing is always prominent in these cases.

Posterior enhancement occurs because the TGC (time gain compensation) is excessive for the low attenuation in the cyst though it is correct for the normal surrounding tissues (see Ch. 1). Enhancement also occurs posterior to many solid tumours, but the enhancement behind cysts is usually more marked in proportion to their size.

Fig. 6.1
Typical simple cyst
The complete absence of internal echoes, the strong posterior enhancement, the oval shape with a thin, smooth wall and edge shadows are typical features of a simple cyst.

ES: edge shadow

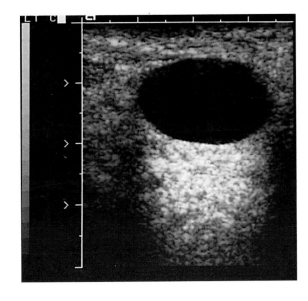
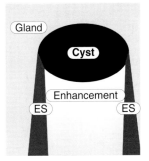

Cysts are usually oval or round in shape. Small cysts tend to be round and become oval as they enlarge (Fig. 6.2), the shape being determined by their tension and by the adjacent glandular structures. Tense cysts are spherical and compress the surrounding structures (Fig. 6.3.a), perhaps accounting for the pain or discomfort they commonly cause. Flaccid cysts are usually flat but may assume a variety of shapes because they extend into the less rigid areas in the breast as they follow the paths of least resistance (Fig. 6.3.b). Small elongated cysts may be difficult to differentiate from dilated ducts but this is clinically unimportant because both are components of benign breast changes.

The typical smooth, thin wall of a cyst is an important feature in the differentiation from other pathologies which have cystic areas, such as necrotic tumours, abscesses or intracystic tumours. Although cysts usually have an epithelial lining histologically, this is only a few cells thick so that the walls themselves are not defined as more than a line on ultrasound.

Fig. 6.2
Round and oval simple cysts
a. A rounded shape is common in cysts smaller than 1 cm in diameter. The typical features that allow a confident diagnosis of a simple cyst are shown. The glandular tissue immediately anterior to this cyst is smoothly compressed, also a benign feature.
b. Cysts tend to become oval as they enlarge. The echo-free contents, thin wall, posterior enhancement and edge shadows are typical features of a simple cyst.

ES: edge shadow
GI: mammary gland
PE: posterior enhancement
RMS: retromammary space
SCF: subcutaneous fat

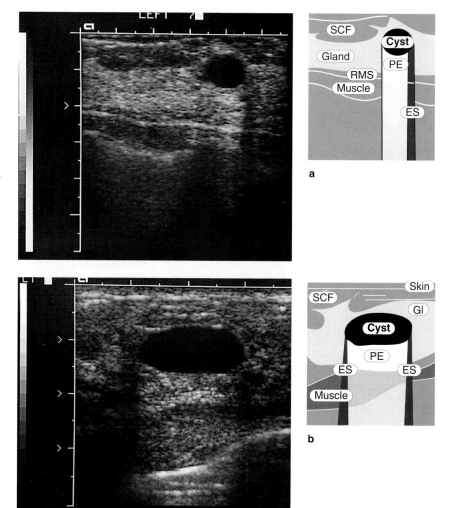

Fig. 6.3
Tense and flaccid cysts
a. Round cysts of this size are relatively uncommon; the round shape implies that the cyst is tense. Such cysts are more often symptomatic.
b. Flattened cysts, such as this example, are not under tension and so are readily compressed under probe pressure. Despite their large size, they are usually impalpable and are generally asymptomatic, being incidental findings on mammograms or ultrasound.

ES: edge shadows
GI: mammary gland
PE: posterior enhancement
RMS: retromammary space
SCF: subcutaneous fat

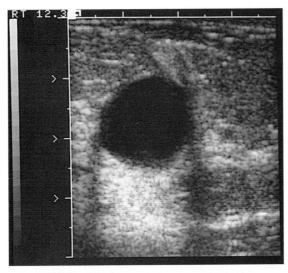

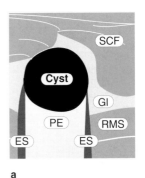

a

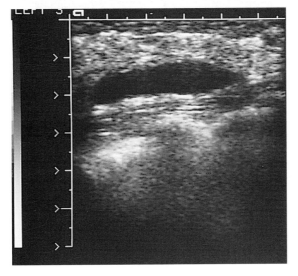

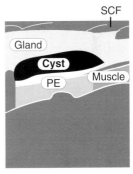

b

When two or more cysts fuse, lobulated spaces are formed (Fig. 6.4.a). Portions of the residual septa may persist as linear sheets extending partway into the cyst (Fig. 6.4.b); they must be differentiated from true proliferative projections (which suggest intracystic papillomas or intracystic carcinomas) which have more obvious and irregular solid components compared with the fragile membranes of septa. Slight irregularity of a cyst wall may result when a cyst is partly emptied, either spontaneously or following needle aspiration (Fig. 6.5).

Fig. 6.4
Lobulated cysts
a. Two lobulated cysts in a multicystic breast, probably formed by fusion of adjacent cysts.
b. The cyst on the right has an incomplete septum; it was formed by partial fusion of two adjacent cysts. The remaining septum (★) is smooth and thin. There is no evidence of an intracystic papillary tumour.

ES: edge shadow
GI: mammary gland
PE: posterior enhancement
SCF: subcutaneous fat
SL: superficial layer of the superficial fascia

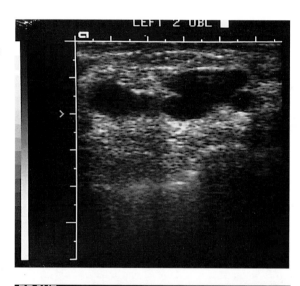
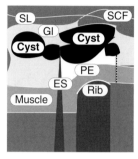

a

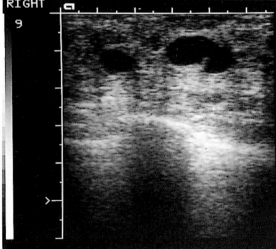
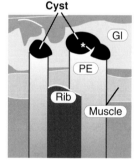

b

Edge shadows are seen with many masses which have smooth margins and are not of diagnostic importance; they must be distinguished from true attenuative shadows, which are a suspicious feature.

On adequate probe pressure, almost all cysts are compressible, except those that are very tense (Fig. 6.6). Mobility is not as obvious as with fibroadenomas because cysts remain attached to the ductal structures from which they originated.

Doppler never shows vessels within a cyst (Plate C.11). The vasculature around a cyst is not usually apparent; occasional exceptions are presumably due to an inflammatory response to leaked cyst fluid or to haemorrhage following needling.

Fig. 6.5
Cyst after aspiration
A follow-up ultrasound was performed after cyst aspiration in this patient. A simple cyst was seen on the previous ultrasound but, after the aspiration, the cyst developed an atypical appearance with an irregular shape, presumably due to haemorrhage. Scanning after aspiration may lead to misinterpretation.

ES: edge shadow
GI: mammary gland
PE: posterior enhancement
SCF: subcutaneous fat

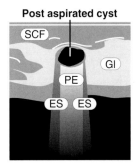

Post aspirated cyst

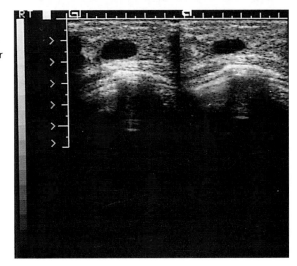

Fig. 6.6
Compression test
Cysts are usually easily compressible as can be demonstrated by transducer pressure.

GI: mammary gland.

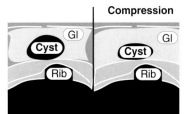

Compression

Artefactual echoes may give an atypical appearance to simple cysts (Table 6.2)[5]. Reverberation is the commonest problem, often seen in superficially located cysts (Fig. 6.7.a); the mechanism is described in Chapter 1. The artefactual echoes appear in the superficial portions of the cyst and, typically, consist of lines parallel to the skin. The distance between the lines is equal to the separation between the paired structures which cause the artefact, usually the skin surface and the anterior wall of the cyst. Use of a stand-off, or simply changing the depth of the cyst by light probe pressure, may solve the problem (Fig. 6.7.b,c).

Table 6.2	Artefacts producing 'atypical appearances' in a cyst

Reverberation artefacts
Slice thickness artefact
Poor lateral resolution
Noise

Fig. 6.7
Reverberation artefacts
a. In this patient with small breasts (overall thickness of only 1.5 cm), a cyst is inevitably superficial. Its anterior part is occupied by weak linear echoes lying parallel to the skin layer. This parallel line pattern is typical of reverberation artefacts.
b. Reverberation artefacts may disappear on changing probe pressure. Reducing compression by partly lifting the transducer increases the distance between the skin surface and the anterior surface of the cyst and may decrease the reverberation artefact (right).
c. The reverberation artefact in this superficial small cyst (right) disappears when imaged using a stand-off (left). Reverberation artefacts are more obvious when they fall onto anechoic cysts but are masked when superimposed onto the glandular tissue.

ES: edge shadow
GI: mammary gland
PE: posterior enhancement
RMS: retromammary space

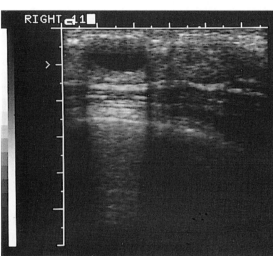

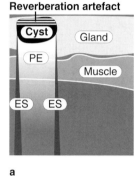

Reverberation artefact

a

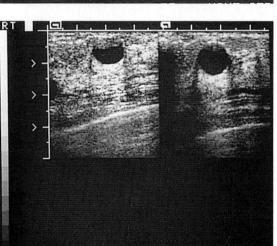

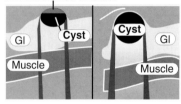

Reverberation artefact

b

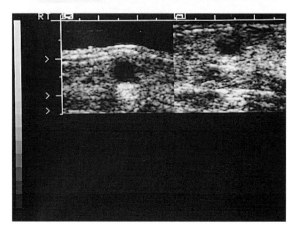

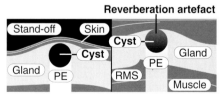

Reverberation artefact

c

The spreading of echoes due to the beam width may blur the margin of a cyst (Fig. 6.8); for best imaging, the lesion should lie in the focal zone. Scattered echoes or side lobes from adjacent tissue may cause apparent echoes in small cysts. Cysts deep in the breast may seem to contain weak internal echoes because the TGC amplifies noise.

Fig. 6.8
Ill-defined margin due to improper setting of focus
This simple cyst has a well-defined margin in (**a**) but the same cyst seems to have an ill-defined margin (★) when the focus is set deep to the lesion (**b**). The focus should be set at the level of the lesion or at its deep border because the ultrasound beam spreads rapidly beyond to the focal zone. More of the scan field can be focused by using multiple focal zones but this reduces the frame rate.

Gl: mammary gland
PE: posterior enhancement.

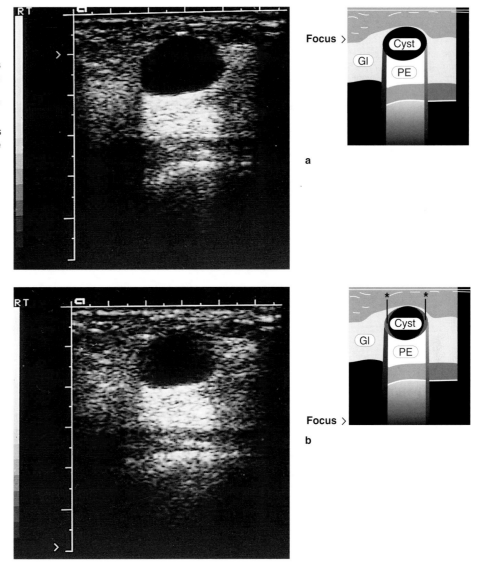

Numerous tiny cysts are typically seen in women on hormone replacement therapy (Fig. 6.9).

COMPLEX CYSTS

The term 'complex cyst' is not a formal pathological classification but is used to describe cysts which deviate in any respect from the appearances of typical ultrasonic cysts. Many of them were previously considered as solid lesions ultrasonographically. As ultrasound has become more widely used, it has become apparent that atypical cysts are common and they frequently cause diagnostic difficulty. Many are impalpable (as many cysts are) and it is important that they are evaluated correctly and distinguished from small carcinomas to avoid unnecessary biopsies. If the view point that 'every ultrasonographically solid lesion needs biopsy' is adopted, then the use of

Fig. 6.9
Multiple cysts
a. In this case the cysts are so numerous that they occupy the entire breast.
b. The cysts in this breast of a 65-year-old woman are small but very numerous. Cysts are uncommon at this age but she was taking hormone replacement therapy (HRT); numerous tiny cysts are more common than large cysts in women on HRT.

ES: edge shadow
Gl: mammary gland
RMS: retromammary space
SCF: subcutaneous fat
SL: superficial layer of the superficial fascia

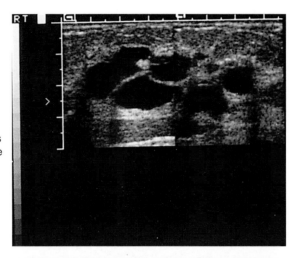

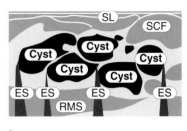

a

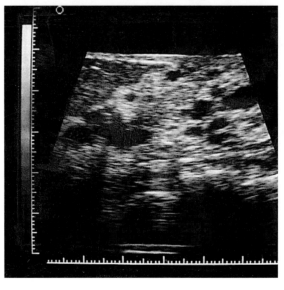

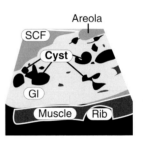

b

ultrasound will increase the frequency of so-called 'benign biopsies' (i.e. those with C0, C1 or C2 cytology). In practice their differentiation from true solid lesions is often difficult and many do need FNAC (fine needle aspiration cytology), best performed under ultrasonic guidance to check that the suspicious lesion is, in fact, punctured. However, there are several reassuring features which are typical of this type of cyst; generally lesions with those appearances can be followed up with ultrasound rather than biopsied immediately.

The causes of complex cysts are listed in Table 6.3. Cysts with scanty internal echoes are usually not a diagnostic problem since all the other typical features remain (Fig. 6.10). The echoes in these lesions usually arise from cell debris that produces cloudy fluid. If movement of these internal echoes is observed (e.g. after repositioning the patient) its fluid nature is confirmed.

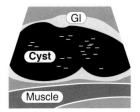

Table 6.3   Causes of complex cysts
Cellular debris
Milk cysts (galactocele)
Concentrated or inspissated material
Bleeding or clot due to needling
Reaction around cysts following leakage
Inflammatory changes

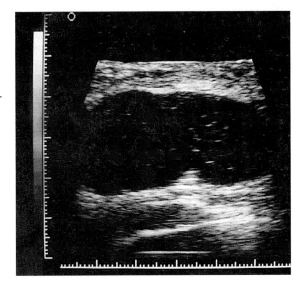

Fig. 6.10
Cyst with sparse internal echoes
Fine internal echoes were demonstrated within this cyst; they moved in a coherent fashion with probe compression and so were considered to be due to debris. Straw-coloured, slightly cloudy fluid was aspirated.

GI: mammary gland

Cysts with posterior shadowing and those showing internal echoes pose a diagnostic problem (Fig. 6.11); a smooth rounded shape, homogeneous internal echoes and displacement or compression of the surrounding tissues without disruption of its structure are benign features. Such lesions usually represent cysts with inspissated or pasty contents, as shown on aspiration; some contain condensed milk. These cysts are usually small and may be impalpable despite their superficial location.

Inspissated material in cysts around the nipple (actually focally dilated ducts or lactiferous sinuses) cause diagnostic difficulty because they mimic intracystic tumours, such as intraductal papillomas; in addition sometimes they are associated with nipple discharge (Fig. 6.12).

Milk of calcium settles under gravity to produce the 'tea-cup' sign on mammograms (Fig. 6.13.a) It is not commonly observed on ultrasound (Fig. 6.13.b) because these cysts are usually very small and the scanty sediment

Fig. 6.11
Complex cysts
'Complex cysts' are those that depart from the classic criteria for a simple cyst. They may, for example, contain internal echoes (**a**, **b**, **c**) or produce posterior shadowing (**b**). The homogeneous internal echoes and round shape with smooth regular contours in these cases are benign appearances but such lesions cannot be diagnosed as cysts with complete confidence and fine needle aspiration is usually required to rule out a small carcinoma. Cysts with these appearances often contain inspissated material.

Gl: mammary gland
RMS: retromammary space
SCF: subcutaneous fat

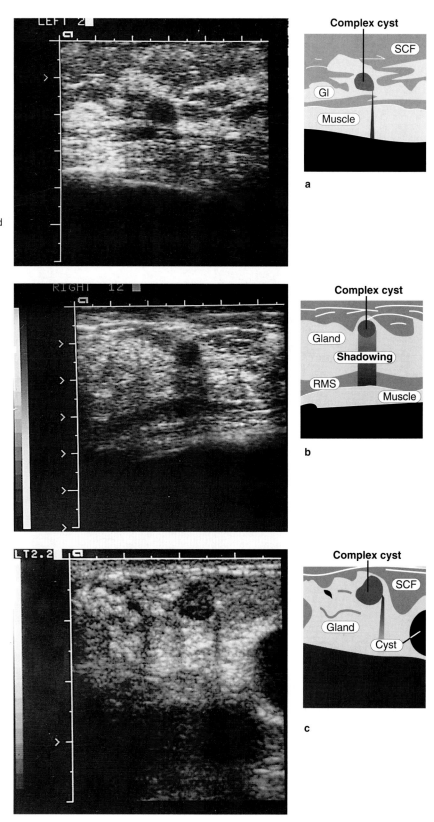

is obscured by the strong echoes from the back of the cyst. Galactoceles are a special pathological category, described separately in this section.

Calcified cysts or old cysts with fibrotic walls also may cast acoustic shadows due to their high attenuation. The former may be confirmed on mammography: they usually have smooth thin walls which are strongly reflective. Calcification occurs more commonly in the wall of oil cysts (see Ch. 8.1).

Fig. 6.12
Inspissated cyst close to the nipple
This 43-year-old woman had a small palpable lump just above the nipple together with nipple discharge. The scan showing a cyst containing an echogenic area is highly suspicious of an intracystic tumour. Very thick, mucoid material was seen in the cyst at surgery and no proliferative change was found histologically. Such echogenic areas are not common in inspissated cysts.

Gl: mammary gland
SCF: subcutaneous cyst

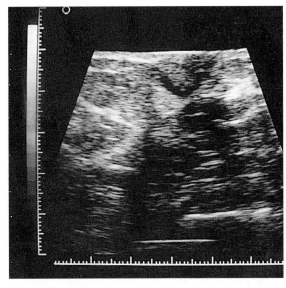
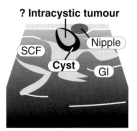

Fig. 6.13
Milk of calcium
a. Curvilinear opacities on the mediolateral mammograms known as the 'tea-cup sign' are formed by a sediment of calcium in small milk cysts. This is an example of benign calcification.
b. The ultrasound equivalent is curvilinear strong echoes that are occasionally observed at the bottom of cysts, probably representing milk of calcium.

ES: edge shadow
Gl: mammary gland

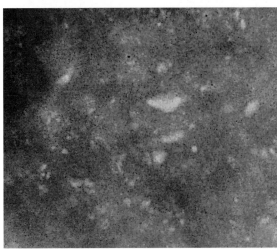

a

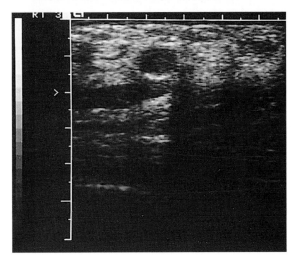
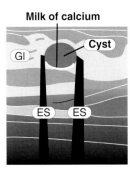

b

Blood clot or bleeding after aspiration of a simple cyst produces confusing appearances (Fig. 6.14), often misinterpreted as an intracystic tumour or as spontaneous bleeding — both highly suspicious of malignancy[6]. Ideally ultrasound should be performed prior to aspiration, otherwise the bleeding may mask small proliferative lesions on the cyst walls. Scanning after needling may result in unnecessary biopsies of iatrogenically complicated cysts.

Thickening of a cyst wall may be caused by inflammatory changes following spontaneous or postaspiration leakage of the contents to the surrounding tissue (Fig.

6.15). These lesions must be differentiated from abscesses, which are usually obvious clinically, and from necrotic tumours, which have more irregular walls.

Because of their confusing appearances, dynamic tests, especially their easy compressibility, are particularly important with complicated cysts. Absence of vessels on a Doppler study also supports the diagnosis.

Fig. 6.14
Cyst post aspiration
A few days before the scan this cyst was aspirated and clear fluid obtained. It now has an echogenic portion with a confusing appearance which probably represents blood clot.

Gl: mammary gland
RMS: retromammary space
SCF: subcutaneous fat
SL: superficial layer of the superficial fascia

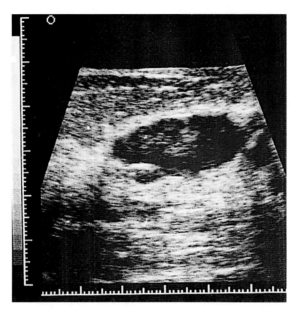

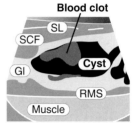

Fig. 6.15
Thick walled cysts

a. This cyst had been aspirated several days before the examination. The wall is thickened but smooth and uniform (★). This was considered to be a reaction from leaked cyst fluid caused by needling. The same appearances may be seen in cysts without a history of aspiration, probably then due to spontaneous leakage. As with all complex cysts, a confident diagnosis is impossible.
b. The centre of this lesion is echo-free, but it has a thick wall. Because of its irregular shape, FNAC was performed under ultrasound guidance; it revealed inflammatory cells, suggesting superinfection.

ES: edge shadow
PE: posterior enhancement
RMS: retromammary space
SCF: subcutaneous fat

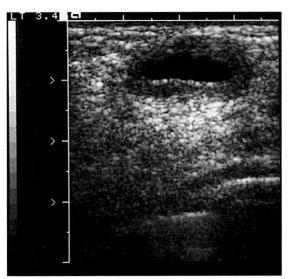

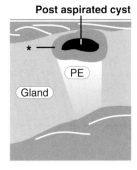

a

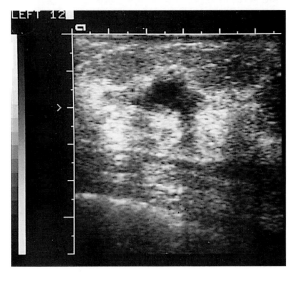

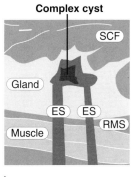

b

GALACTOCELES

A galactocele is a cyst filled with milk that occurs after lactation, most commonly after abrupt artificial suppression. Usually the history is of a painless swelling in the breast developing over a few weeks or months. On palpation galactoceles are indistinguishable from a simple cyst,

though they may be hard if tense. Aspiration usually yields milk and the mass disappears.

Histologically, galactoceles are lined by the normal double layer of breast epithelial and myoepithelial cells, the former not exhibiting apocrine metaplasia but often showing secretory activity.

The ultrasound appearances are more confusing than

Fig. 6.16
Ultrasound of milk
Milk contains echoes because of its fat droplets. This is a scan of full cream milk in a thin walled bag.

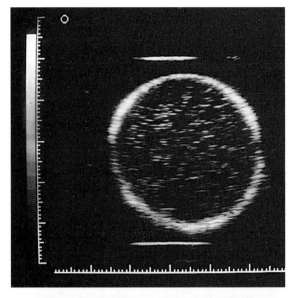

Fig. 6.17
Galactocele
These lesions appeared after stopping nursing. The echo intensity of galactoceles is variable, probably depending on degree of concentration of the milk. They may have the same level of internal echoes as the glandular tissue (which is typically echo-poor in the lactating breast) (**a**, **b**). In these cases, the galactocele may be difficult to detect.

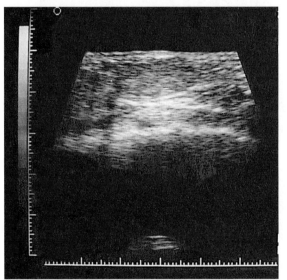

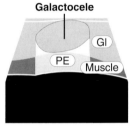

a

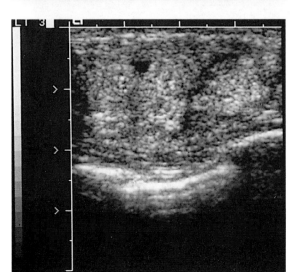

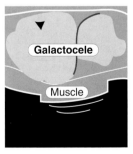

b

the clinical findings. Milk has strong reflectivity because of the fat droplets it contains (Fig. 6.16) and therefore galactoceles often seem solid on ultrasound (Fig. 6.17). They may be oval or lobulated, while the well-circumscribed, smooth margins and homogeneous texture often give an appearance similar to fibroadenomas. Both fibroadenomas and carcinomas may enlarge during pregnancy and may first become palpable after cessation of lactation when the breasts involute and soften. Doppler is helpful in this situation because there are no vessels within a galactocele whereas the surrounding parenchyma is hyperaemic because of lactational activity. Complete lack of vascularity is unusual in carcinomas and even fibroadenomas usually contain a few vessels, especially those stimulated by pregnancy or lactation. Occasionally, a galactocele is difficult to detect at all on ultrasound because its texture is so similar to the surrounding parenchyma of the lactating breast. Dynamic tests, especially scanning during palpation, are useful in revealing such masses and for evaluating their nature.

SEBACEOUS CYSTS

A sebaceous cyst is a retention cyst that follows plugging of the orifice of a sebaceous gland in the skin. They may develop at any site, including the skin of the breast. They are entirely distinct from breast cysts. Because of their superficial location, they are often visible as a nodule within the skin. As well as being palpable, the orifice of the gland is often seen as a small dark punctum on the skin surface.

Pathologically, sebaceous cysts are lined by squamous epithelium and contain large amounts of keratin.

Scanning during palpation is useful. A galactocele may be echo-poor (**c**, **d**). The lobulated echo-poor galactocele in (**c**) has a similar appearance to a fibroadenoma, but its avascular nature on colour Doppler study supported the diagnosis.

ES: edge shadow
GI: mammary gland
PE: posterior enhancement
SCF: subcutaneous fat

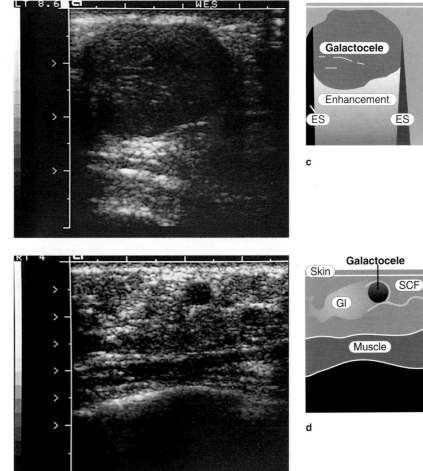

On ultrasound they may appear as almost anechoic areas, similar to true cysts, or as relatively echogenic areas, usually with posterior enhancement (Fig. 6.18). Their most characteristic feature is their superficial location anterior to the superficial layer of the superficial fascia, thus excluding an origin from breast epithelium, and they are attached to the skin. The deeper layers of the skin are often inapparent on the image and the skin is thinned at the site of the sebaceous cyst. Occasionally a small tubular structure is seen between the cyst and the skin surface; this is actually the excretory duct.

Fig. 6.18
Sebaceous cyst
Sebaceous cysts form from sebaceous glands of the skin and therefore are located anterior to the superficial layer of the superficial fascia and are attached to the skin (**a**). A fine connection to the skin orifice may be seen on a magnified scan (**b**).

GI: mammary gland
PE: posterior enhancement
SL: superficial layer of the superficial fascia

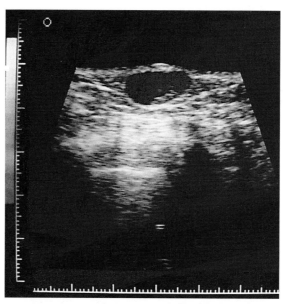
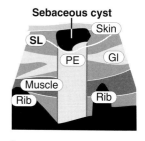

a

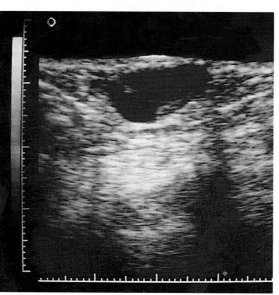
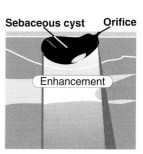

b

REFERENCES

1. S.v.W. Hilton, G.R. Leopold, L.K. Olson, S.A. Willson: Real-time breast sonography: application in 300 consecutive patients. AJR 147; 479–486, 1986.
2. L.W. Bassett, C. Kimme-Smith, L.K. Sutherland, et al: Automated and hand-held breast US: effect on patient management. Radiology 165; 103–108, 1987.
3. J. Jellins, G. Kossoff, T.S. Reeve: Detection and classification of liquid-filled masses in the breast by gray scale echography. Radiology 125; 205–212, 1977.
4. E.A. Sickles, R.A. Filly, P.W. Callen: Benign breast lesions: ultrasound detection and diagnosis. Radiology 151; 467–470, 1984.
5. C. Kimme-Smith, P.A. Rothschild, L.W. Bassett, et al: Ultrasound artifacts affecting the diagnosis of breast masses. Ultrasound Med Biol 14 (suppl 1); 203–210, 1988.
6. W.E. Svensson, E. Tohno, D.O. Cosgrove, T.J. Powles, B. Hussani, A.L. Jones: Effects of fine needle aspiration on the ultrasound appearances of the breast. Radiology 185; 709–711, 1992.

6.2 BENIGN BREAST CHANGE

CLINICAL FEATURES

Benign breast change is a very common problem that causes much confusion both clinically, mammographically, ultrasonographically and histologically. There is much debate about its precise identity and even as to its existence as a clinicopathological entity.

Many terms have been used to describe the condition, including 'chronic cystic mastitis'[7], 'chronic mastitis', 'chronic cystic disease'[8], 'mammary dysplasia', 'fibroadenosis', 'fibrocystic mastopathy', 'cystic hyperplasia', 'mazoplasia' and 'mastopathy'. These terms reflect the different and varied morphological components. While 'fibrocystic disease' is one of the most commonly used terms, especially in the United States, 'benign breast change' is preferred in this text since the fibrous and cystic components are not invariably present and there is no definite evidence that any of the changes represents disease (see below). 'ANDI' (aberration of normal development and involution) is a recently introduced term[9] which has found favour in many centres.

Evidence that the process may not represent a disease process at all comes from autopsy studies[10]. In one series a 19% incidence of gross cystic disease in normal breasts was found at postmortem examination; when microscopic proliferation, cystic disease or apocrine epithelial changes were included, the incidence rose to 53%[8]. On the other hand, Vorherr states that "fibrocystic breast disease is not a 'harmless nondisease' but a distinct clinical entity that requires treatment to bring about relief to the patient, to reduce the incidence of breast surgical procedures, and the risk of breast cancer"[11]. In general, whether benign breast change represents a pathological or a physiological process is a quantitative rather than a qualitative question; when the changes cause clinical, mammographic or ultrasonic problems, they may properly be called a 'disease'.

Another problem is whether benign breast change is associated with an increased risk of developing breast carcinoma. Certain types of histological change seem to be associated with a slight or moderately increased risk[12], as is discussed further under 'pathological features'.

Little is known about the aetiology and epidemiology of benign breast change, partly because of confusion about definitions and terminology. It is considered to be hormonally induced, possibly by oestrogen predominance over progesterone or by persistent exposure to oestrogens. Oestrogens stimulate proliferative changes in the breast with growth of periductal stroma and of ducts while progesterone counteracts these proliferative effects and also promotes lobular development. Deficiency of the corpus luteum or anovulation have been reported to be common in patients with benign breast change (the 'luteal deficiency hypothesis')[13] and progesterones are used in treatment. The effects of oral contraceptives are also controversial[14], but there is evidence of different effects on different histological components: a reduced incidence of cysts and blunt duct adenosis with an increased incidence of lacta-tional foci and no change in the incidence of intraductal hyperplasia have been reported[15].

Ideally the clinical, ultrasound and mammographic features should be correlated with histology but, in benign breast change, typical cases do not need biopsy, so this is not usually possible. Furthermore, the pathological changes are often microscopic and a variety of features are often intermingled in the same specimen, adding to the problems of understanding.

The clinical features can be divided into four groups: mastalgia, nodularity, discrete lumps and nipple discharge, which may coexist in any combination. Typically mastalgia and nodularity vary through the menstrual cycle, being worse in the premenstrual phase. Both are probably due to a hormonally controlled increase in blood supply to the breast and intramammary oedema. The texture of the nodularity is often likened to a 'bag of peas'. The margins of the individual nodules are usually ill-defined. Discrete lumps are most commonly due to cysts though any other changes may cause a mass if one portion of the breast is particularly severely affected. Such masses need to be distinguished from true tumours, especially carcinomas. Nipple discharge is not a common symptom; when it occurs, multiple ducts are often involved and the discharge has a variety of appearances including brown, green, blue or milky yellow fluid (see Ch. 5.3).

PATHOLOGICAL FEATURES

A wide variety of epithelial and stromal alterations may be encountered singly or in any combination. The use of the term 'benign breast change', or any of the other all-embracing terms listed above, has three major disadvantages:

1. There is no evidence that all changes share the same aetiology — indeed, there is evidence to the contrary (see earlier)
2. Each of the changes produces different clinical manifestations, e.g. cysts are rounded fluctuant swellings, major duct ectasia may produce discharge from the nipple
3. Not all changes have the same implications for the patient's management, particularly the atypical intraductal and intralobular hyperplasias, which carry an increased risk of malignancy.

Changes may take the form of dilatation of acini within terminal duct lobular units to produce cysts or within interlobular ducts to produce duct ectasia. The pathology of these two changes is described on pages 104 and 136. Various forms of adenosis may be observed, usually only microscopic in size. Unqualified, this term is used to describe enlargement of TDLUs without structural or cytological abnormalities. In some cases, isolated enlarged TDLUs may show secretory changes identical to those seen in pregnancy and lactation when they are known as 'lactational foci' (Plate P.6.2). Blunt duct adenosis is a form of organoid lobular hypertrophy composed of two-layered epithelial tubules embedded in specialised stroma. The tubules show a minor degree of cystic dilatation and there is hypertrophy of the lining epithelial cells which become columnar with large hyperchromatic nuclei (Plate P.6.3).

Sclerosing adenosis is a form of lobular enlargement in which the acini are increased in number and acquire distorted, spiky, infiltrative outlines, often accompanied by obliteration of the lumina (Plate P.6.4). Although benign, the epithelium may infiltrate the surrounding stroma, including nerves and blood vessels. The lobular architecture is retained, however. Sclerosing adenosis is usually of microscopic size but coalescence of several adjacent involved lobules may produce a palpable mass.

A radial scar is also a common benign lesion in which the epithelium may show a tendency to infiltrate the surrounding stroma. It has a characteristic architecture with a central fibroelastotic zone from which radiate out tubular structures lined either by hyperplastic or normal two-layered epithelium (Plate P.6.5). Rarely the epithelium may show atypical hyperplasia or even in situ carcinoma. Radial scars are usually less than 1 cm in maximum diameter. When they are larger, they are generally known as 'complex sclerosing lesions' which form nodular masses of sclerosing adenosis with papillary proliferation around the periphery (Plate P.6.6). Macroscopically, radial scars and complex sclerosing lesions may form hard irregular masses that simulate carcinomas.

There is no evidence that any of the changes described so far are associated with an increased risk of developing carcinoma. This is not the case, however, with various forms of intraluminal cellular proliferation. In hyperplasia of the usual type there is intraluminal proliferation of epithelial cells, myoepithelial cells, lymphocytes and macrophages (Plate P.6.7). In the more florid cases, the ductal structures may be markedly distended but the lesions are rarely of macroscopic size. Cellular composition and cytological appearances are the main features that distinguish hyperplasia from in situ carcinoma. The distinction is usually straightforward but there are borderline cases in which some, but not all, features of malignancy are present. Such cases are usually classified as 'atypical hyperplasia' of which two forms are recognised: atypical ductal hyperplasia (Plate P.6.8) and atypical lobular hyperplasia (Plate P.6.9). Despite their names, both predominantly affect the TDLUs. Atypical lobular hyperplasia is distinguished by the presence of characteristic small rounded cells, similar to those found in in situ and infiltrating lobular carcinomas. Atypical ductal hyperplasia, on the other hand, has a much more variable appearance like ductal carcinoma in situ (see page 178). A large number of clinical studies has related the various forms of hyperplasia to the subsequent development of a carcinoma. The findings have been somewhat conflicting but the balance of evidence points to an association between these lesions and an increased risk of developing carcinoma. A consensus statement was issued by a large gathering of eminent American pathologists in 1986. At this meeting, it was accepted that papillary or solid hyperplasia is associated with a slightly increased risk (1.5 to 2 times) and atypical ductal or lobular hyperplasia associated with a moderately increased risk (5 times) of developing carcinoma[12].

ULTRASOUND FEATURES

The role of ultrasound for the patients with benign breast change is twofold: to diagnose underlying palpable abnormalities as benign (to exclude malignancy) and to detect coexistent carcinomas in diffuse lumpy or mammographically dense breasts. Carcinomas have the same appearances in normal breasts as in those with benign breast change but precancerous lesions, such as atypical hyperplasia, cannot be identified. The appearances of breast carcinomas are described in the chapter on malignant diseases; in this chapter the general features of benign breast change are described.

Table 6.4 shows the approximate correlations between the clinical, ultrasound and histological features.

Ultrasound is usually not indicated for mastalgia, especially when periodic, unless it is accompanied by other features. Because pain is so subjective, there is no specific abnormality on ultrasound but the glandular tissue is usually thick in patients with mastalgia, though of normal texture.

In generalised nodularity, especially in large breasts, evaluation of each suspicious region and to exclude carcinoma by palpation is difficult and time consuming, though skilled clinicians achieve remarkably high success

Table 6.4	Correlation between clinical, ultrasound and histological features in benign breast changes	
Clinical features	**Ultrasound features**	**Histology**
Mastalgia	Normal	(Biopsy not usually indicated)
	Thickened gland with normal architecture	
Nodularity	Thickened gland with normal architecture	
	Multiple cysts	Cysts Apocrine metaplasia
	Diffuse or multiple architectural changes 'Mottled pattern' Echo-poor gland	Non-specific*
	Shadowing	Fibrosis
Mass	Focal thickening of the gland with normal architecture	Non-specific*
	Cyst, dilated duct	Cyst, duct ectasia
	Focal architectural change	Non-specific*
	Mass	(Sclerosing) adenosis
Nipple discharge	Dilated ducts	Duct ectasia

* 'Non-specific' refers to the whole spectrum of benign breast change, including various forms of adenosis, apocrine metaplasia, cysts, duct ectasia, fibrosis and ductal or lobular hyperplasia.

rates. In these women mammograms often show dense or multinodular tissue and are of little help. On ultrasound, however, the gland is thickened but often of normal texture or contains multiple cysts. In these cases the probability of carcinoma is extremely low. Architectural change may be seen either diffusely or multifocally; those appearances are described later in this section, but their severity on ultrasound is poorly correlated with the extent of palpable abnormalities.

Even when there is a localised lump, ultrasound often shows no lesion or merely either localised thickening of the gland (Fig. 6.19) or normal glandular tissue with a nodular surface. Cysts as a cause of lumps can be proven by aspiration, but they may lie deep in the glandular tissue where aspiration is difficult. (The ultrasound features of cysts are described in Chapter 6.1.) Cysts that are typical on ultrasound do not need aspiration except to relieve pain or if there is concern that they may mask a tumour.

Aspiration can be performed under ultrasound guidance, if indicated.

Thickened glands may be homogeneously echogenic with a normal texture but they often show diffuse or multiple architectural changes. The histological correlates of these changes are non-specific, usually consisting of a mixture of many changes. Differentiation from other lesions, especially carcinomas, necessitates careful scanning with attention to subtle details. Their distribution is characteristic: they are usually bilateral and multiple. Although the changes may be extensive and the margins of these lesions are often poorly defined, merging gradually into normal tissues, secondary features of malignancy, such as invasion of fatty tissue or interruption of the glandular surface, are not seen. The normal ductal structures of the glandular layer pass through these regions of altered architecture rather than being interrupted or deviated, as is typical of true masses.

Fig. 6.19
Focal glandular thickening causing a palpable mass
The glandular tissue has involuted and been replaced by fatty tissue through most of the breast. At the site of the palpable mass, the glandular tissue is thickened and homogeneously echogenic, a normal appearance.

PMiM: pectoralis minor muscle
PMjM: pectoralis major muscle
RMS: retromammary space
SCF: subcutaneous fat
SL: superficial layer of the superficial fascia

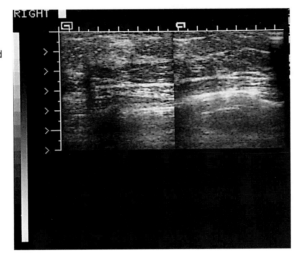

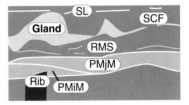

The commonest architectural change is the appearance of small echo-poor regions in the glandular tissue (Fig. 6.20.a). Seen in long axis, these are actually tubular structures radiating from the nipple (see Ch. 3.5). This change may be seen in asymptomatic subjects, especially in young women, and is considered to be a normal variation, but is often present in lumpy or nodular breasts and is sometimes focal, especially in nodular areas (Fig. 6.20.b). These echo-poor areas can be distinguished from simple dilated ducts because they are not echo-free. Ueno termed this appearance the 'mottled pattern'[16]. The precise histological correlation is unknown, but ultrasonically they appear to correspond to changes in the periductal regions; periductal fibrosis or epithelial proliferation are suggested causes. Occasionally, smaller echo-free areas are seen at the centre of these structures, probably representing the lumina of the ducts themselves (Fig. 6.20.c).

Other architectural changes include low level echoes

Fig. 6.20
The 'mottled pattern'
a. The glandular tissue is thickened and contains numerous echo-poor foci. This 'mottled pattern' is a normal variant but is more often seen in lumpy breasts. The presence of low level echoes distinguishes them from dilated ducts. These structures probably consist of ducts of normal calibre with associated periductal changes.
b. A 'mottled pattern' (M) may also be evident in normal mammary gland (N). It may be focal, especially in nodular or lumpy areas.
c. When imaged radially, the echo-poor regions of the mottled pattern are seen to be linear structures corresponding with the lie of the ducts. Occasionally anechoic areas are seen within these linear structures, probably representing the lumina of the ducts themselves.

GI: mammary gland
IS: interface shadow from the Cooper's ligament
SCF: subcutaneous fat

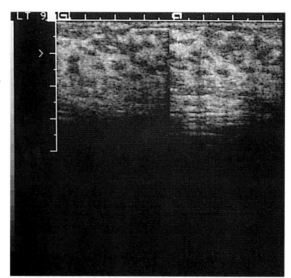
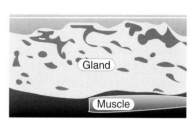

a

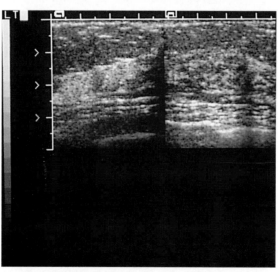
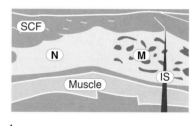

b

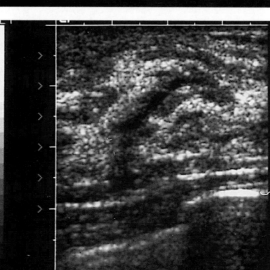
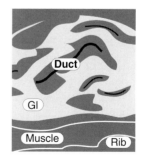

c

from the gland and diffuse shadowing (Fig. 6.21). The echogenicity of the gland may be similar to that of the fatty tissue but is never as echo-poor as the nidus of a carcinoma. Shadowing in benign breast change is probably due to fibrosis, just as in carcinomas and scars. (This shadowing must be distinguished from the fine edge shadows from ligaments or fat/gland interfaces, which are of no diagnostic significance.) Diffuse or multiple shadowing is unusual in a carcinoma and, while rarely a carcinoma may only produce shadowing and no mass, these are usually large, diffusely invasive lesions that are clinically obvious. Extensive shadowing due to fibrosis may also be observed in patients with long standing insulin-dependent diabetes, a curious change known as 'diabetic fibrous mastopathy'[17] (Fig. 6.22). Autoimmunity or cross-linkage with increased collagen production are suggested mechanisms[18,19].

Fig. 6.21
Architectural change
a. Echo-poor gland. Part of the gland of this breast (EP) is diffusely echo-poor, while elsewhere the gland shows a mottled pattern (M). The echo-poor portion has a similar echogenicity to the fatty tissue but can be distinguished from it because of its convex surface. An echo-poor gland is not a common finding but is sometimes seen in nodular breasts.
b. Diffuse shadowing due to benign breast change. In this case shadowing is seen from a wide region of the gland. Though it originates from the glandular tissue itself, there is no nidus as would occur with a tumour. The shadowing is probably caused by fibrosis but these changes must be distinguished from a diffuse breast carcinoma. Since the texture of the glandular tissue is preserved within the shadowing area, this appearance is unlikely to be due to a carcinoma.

RMS: retromammary space
SCF: subcutaneous fat

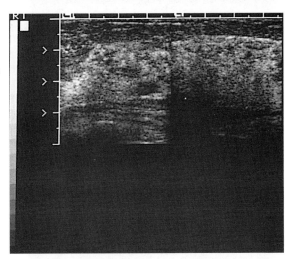
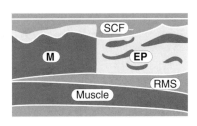
a

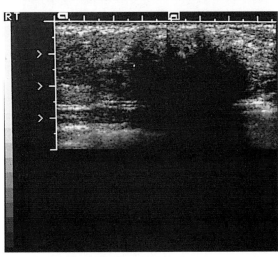
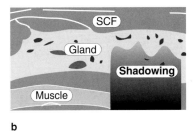
b

Fig. 6.22
Diabetic fibrous disease
A hard lump was felt in the right breast of this 34-year-old woman with a 20-year history of insulin-dependent diabetes mellitus. On ultrasound there is a wide area of marked shadowing which precludes evaluation of the internal texture. Although this area is very extensive, the gland retains its normal cone shape and there are no secondary signs of malignancy, such as increased echogenicity of the subcutaneous fat.

SCF: subcutaneous fat

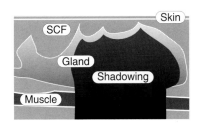

Focal thickening of the glandular tissue without architectural distortion, cysts or dilated ducts are readily defined on ultrasound and this solves the question as to the cause of the thickening. Focal architectural changes are usually identical to the diffuse or multiple changes described above, but, if they are solitary or very marked, careful evaluation is needed to differentiate them from malignancy. Focal benign breast change does not have a nidus and, if a 'mottled pattern' or tiny cysts are seen in this area, the lesion is unlikely to be a tumour because tumours destroy or displace both normal tissue and benign changes (Fig. 6.23). Similarly, if ductal structures can be defined traversing the 'mass', malignancy is very unlikely. Shadowing is often associated with focal architectural changes and this makes the lesion seem suspicious. Where the evaluation of the centre of the 'lesion' is difficult because of strong shadowing, compressing with the transducer is helpful since benign tissues can be com-

Fig. 6.23
Focal architectural change due to benign breast change
a. The glandular tissue is focally thickened and echo-poor; furthermore this area causes shadowing, a worrying feature. However, a 'mottled pattern' is seen in this region, suggesting that the texture of the glandular tissue is preserved. The D:W ratio of this 'lesion' is small and there is no break of the glandular surface. The overall appearance suggests benign breast change: only stromal fibrosis was found on histology.
b. One part of the glandular tissue has shadowing, a suspicious feature. However, on the magnified image (**c**) there is no mass in this area and there are small tubular structures (★) in the shadowing region with the same pattern as in the surrounding glandular tissue. This is a key feature in differentiating shadowing due to benign breast change from that of tumours.

GI: mammary gland
RMS: retromammary space
SCF: subcutaneous fat

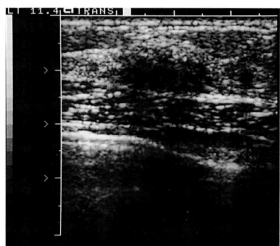

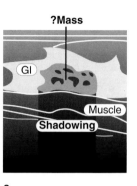

a

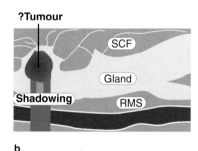

b

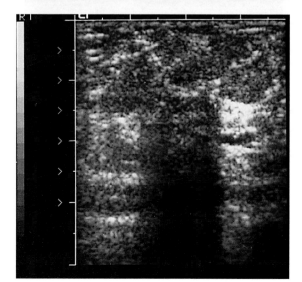

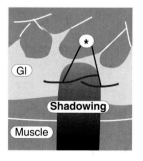

c

pressed, rendering the shadowing less prominent and allowing evaluation of the internal structure (Fig. 6.24). If a nidus is still seen after compression, the lesion should be biopsied.

Breast carcinomas without a mass, especially those detected because of microcalcification on the mammogram, may be seen as focal architectural changes or as shadowing without a nidus. These uncommon carcinomas are difficult to diagnose by ultrasound alone. If severe changes are seen in only one part of the breast, biopsy is indicated; ductal or lobular hyperplasia is often found (Fig. 6.25), though most such abnormalities are caused by focal benign breast changes.

Fig. 6.24
Compression of the shadowing area
A shadowing area lying close to the nipple (left half of scan) raises the suspicion of malignancy. However, it almost disappears on probe compression (right half of scan), revealing glandular tissue with a normal texture and no echo-poor nidus. The cause of this type of shadowing is not fully understood but its disappearance on compression may be because the soft non-malignant parenchyma thins under probe pressure.

RMS: retromammary space

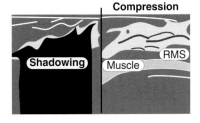

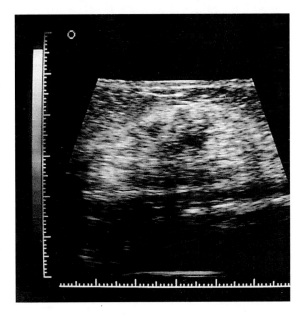

Fig. 6.25
Focal architectural change — atypical lobular hyperplasia
A part of the gland is thickened with an altered texture but there is no clear nidus. Atypical lobular hyperplasia was found on histology. Atypia is a histological diagnosis and cannot be made clinically or on imaging. Lesions with such severe architectural change often contain atypical proliferative changes which carry an increased risk of malignancy.

Gl: mammary gland
SCF: subcutaneous fat
RMS: retromammary space

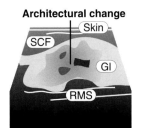

Focal masses are not a common feature of benign breast change but adenosis may form echo-poor masses, usually smaller than 1 cm in diameter. They are regular in shape with no distal enhancement, thus overall resembling fibroadenomas, though they are less mobile. These lesions are usually impalpable. Sclerosing adenosis occasionally forms a palpable mass and is difficult to differentiate from carcinoma on ultrasound, especially as it produces shadowing and has an irregular shape with ill-defined margins (Fig. 6.26).

Dilated ducts are very common findings on ultrasound (Fig. 6.27.a). They may form a palpable mass in the sub-areolar region (Fig. 6.27.b) or be associated with nipple discharge, but often are asymptomatic. Multiple dilated ducts radiating from the nipple are commonly seen in older (postmenopausal) women and they often contain scanty internal echoes due to cell debris, fatty acid crystals or cells (especially foam cells, i.e. macrophages phagocytosing fat). 'Duct ectasia' is a special clinical category in which the duct dilatation is complicated by an

Fig. 6.26
Sclerosing adenosis
A discrete mass with an irregular margin, heterogeneous internal echoes and heterogeneous shadowing raises the suspicion of a breast carcinoma, although there are no invasive appearances such as a halo or interruption of the glandular surface; the histology of this lesion was a mixture of sclerosing adenosis and fibrosis. The fibrous components of sclerosing adenosis may cause shadowing and, especially, the ill-defined margins when the adjacent tissues are involved; they are very difficult to differentiate from a carcinoma on ultrasound.

Gl: mammary gland
SCF: subcutaneous fat

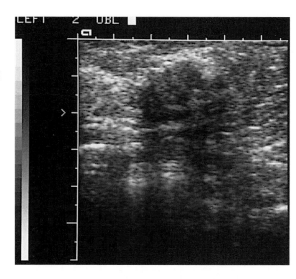
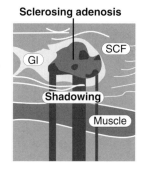

Fig. 6.27
Duct dilatation
a. Some of the multiple dilated ducts converging onto the nipple contain weak echoes because of debris, acid crystals or foam cells. Duct dilatation is encountered in elderly women, whereas other benign breast changes are common in premenopausal women. Duct dilatation may lead to nipple retraction because of fibrosis resulting from inflammation around the ducts.
b. Dilated ducts may form a palpable mass around the nipple. This cystic area behind the areola is different from the usual pattern of a cyst because of its branching 'tree-like' shape. The duct lumina are not completely echo-free.

Gl: mammary gland
SCF: subcutaneous fat
RMS: retromammary space

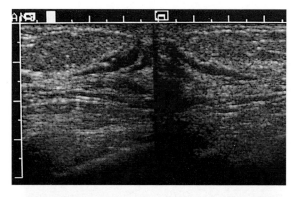
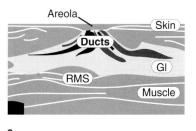

a

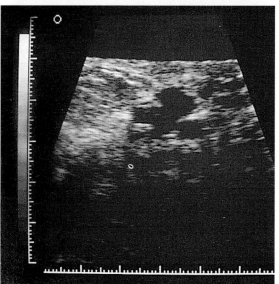
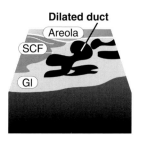

b

inflammatory process (see Ch. 7). The echoes in the dilated ducts are usually diffuse and weak and must be differentiated from true solid tissue (e.g. intraductal proliferative lesions) which are usually focal with strong echoes. The differential diagnoses of dilated ducts are described in Chapter 5.3.

The mammographic appearances in benign breast change are often non-specific; density or nodularity are commonly reported[20] and ultrasound is useful in the detection of lesions hidden in these densities. Radial scars appear as stellate lesions on mammograms; they cannot usually be detected on ultrasound[21] and, because some 'stellate' carcinomas are missed on ultrasound, their management depends on the mammographic features. When seen, radial scars have an irregular shape, very similar to carcinomas (Fig. 6.28). Because microcalcifications in benign breast change are not associated with masses, but are located in lobules or terminal ducts or in the fibrotic stroma, they are difficult to detect on ultrasound. Histological atypia may be found in these lesions; biopsy is indicated according to the mammographic features.

On Doppler, no increase in vascularity is usually demonstrable in benign breast change even in gross cases (Plate C.9) unless complicated by true inflammation, such as in duct ectasia[22]. This negative finding is very useful for differentiation from those breast carcinomas that do not form a mass, where increased blood supply is an important finding. Since breast vascularity has a wide range of variation, comparison with the opposite breast may be useful because benign breast change often occurs bilaterally and the Doppler features are symmetrical. The blood supply to the breast changes through the menstrual cycle with increased flow during the luteal phase[23]; whether this relates to cyclic mastalgia remains unproven.

Fig. 6.28
Radial scar
a. This echo-poor lesion has a very irregular shape, raising the suspicion of malignancy. Histologically a radial scar was found.
b. The palpable mass in this 22-year-old woman has an irregular shape with a high D:W ratio. The appearances are not those of a fibroadenoma, the commonest cause of breast lumps at this age. Malignancy could not be excluded. Histologically this lesion was a 'complex sclerosing lesion', a complex form of radial scar.

Gl: mammary gland

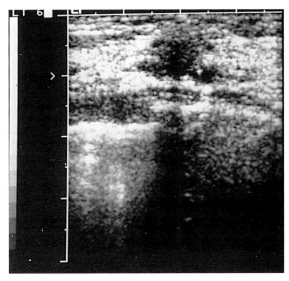
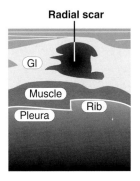

a

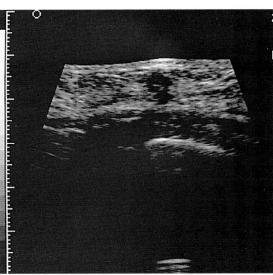
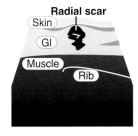

b

REFERENCES

7. F.W. Foote, F.W. Stewart: Comparative studies of cancerous versus noncancerous breasts. Ann Surg 121; 6–53, 1945.

8. V.K. Frantz, J.W. Pickren, G.W. Melcher, H. Auchincloss: Incidence of chronic cystic disease in so-called 'normal breasts' — a study based on 225 postmortem examinations. Cancer 4; 762–783, 1951.

9. L.E. Hughes, R.E. Mansel, D.J.T. Webster: Aberrations of normal development and involution (ANDI): a new perspective on pathogenesis and nomenclature of benign breast disorders. Lancet ii; 1316–1319, 1987.

10. S.M. Love, R.S. Gelman, W. Silen: Fibrocystic 'disease' of the breast — a nondisease? N Engl J Med 307; 1010–1014, 1982.

11. H. Vorherr: Fibrocystic breast disease: pathophysiology, pathomorphology, clinical picture, and management. Am J Obstet Gynecol 154; 161–179, 1986

12. Consensus Meeting: Is 'fibrocystic disease' of the breast precancerous? Arch Pathol Lab Med 110; 171–173, 1986.

13. R. Sitruk-Ware, N. Sterkers, P. Mauvais-Jarvis: Benign breast disease I: Hormonal investigation. Obstet Gynecol 53; 457–460, 1979.

14. H. Ory, P. Cole, B. MacMahon, R. Hoover: Oral contraceptives and reduced risk of benign breast diseases. N Engl J Med 294; 419–422, 1976.

15. G. Hulman, P. Trowbridge, G.N. Taylor, C.E.D. Chilvers, J.P. Sloane: Oral contraceptive use and histopathology of cancerous breasts in young women. Journal of Pathology 167; 407–411, 1992.

16. E. Ueno, E. Tohno, Y. Hirano, et al: Ultrasound diagnosis of breast cancer. J Med Imaging 6; 178–188, 1986.

17. W.I.H. Gartstin, Z.K. Aufmann, M.J. Michell, M. Baum: Fibrous mastopathy in insulin dependent diabetes. Clin Radiol 44; 89–91, 1991.

18. N.G. Soler, R. Khardori: Fibrous disease of the breast, thyroiditis, and cheiroarthropathy in type I diabetes mellitus. Lancet i; 193–194, 1984.

19. B.F. Byrd, W.H. Hartmann, L.S. Graham, H.H. Hogle: Mastopathy in insulin-dependent diabetics. Ann Surg 205; 529–532, 1987.

20. Proposals by the Breast Group of the Royal College of Radiologists: Radiological nomenclature in benign breast change. Clin Radiol 40; 374–379, 1989.

21. J.S. Mitnick, M.F. Vazquez, M.N. Harris, D.F. Roses: Differentiation of radial scar from scirrhous carcinoma of the breast: mammographic–pathologic correlation. Radiology 173; 697–700, 1989.

22. D.O. Cosgrove, J.C. Bamber, J.B. Davey, et al: Colour Doppler signals from breast tumours, work in progress. Radiology 176; 175–180, 1990.

23. M. Sambrook, J.C. Bamber, H. Minasian, C.R. Hill: Ultrasonic Doppler study of the hormonal response of blood flow in the normal human breast. Ultrasound Med Biol 13: 121–129, 1987.

6.3 GYNAECOMASTIA

CLINICAL FEATURES

Gynaecomastia is enlargement of the epithelial and specialised stromal tissues of the breast in the male; breast enlargement due to fat deposition (often accompanied by obesity) is not included. The condition is unilateral in some 75% of cases and about 25% regress spontaneously. Gynaecomastia is clinically important because it may be mistaken for a carcinoma and because it may be the consequence of another disease[24].

Because carcinoma of the male breast itself is uncommon (accounting for less than 1% of all breast carcinomas), the combination of gynaecomastia and carcinoma is very rare. There is no evidence that gynaecomastia is a premalignant condition but it is important to exclude carcinoma as a cause of the breast enlargement, especially when it is asymmetrical or unilateral.

The causes of gynaecomastia are listed in Table 6.5[25]. Gynaecomastia resulting from physiological hormonal changes occurs in the neonate, during puberty and in senescence (due to maternal oestrogens or to an imbalance between androgen and oestrogen levels). Oestrogen treatment of prostatic carcinoma is the commonest cause of gynaecomastia overall. Many other drugs, such as antihypertensives, digitalis, antidepressants and cytotoxics may also cause gynaecomastia through a variety of mechanisms[26,27]. Idiopathic and drug-induced gynaecomastia is particularly likely to be unilateral.

The physical findings are either a localised firm, mobile discoid plaque or a more generalised swelling that resembles the adolescent female breast in appearance and consistency. A minor degree of physical discomfort, such as pain or tenderness, often accompany the change. Rarely nipple discharge may occur.

PATHOLOGICAL FEATURES

The histological changes of gynaecomastia have been divided into active, inactive and intermediate phases[28,29]. In the active phase, the ducts are increased in number and may show some dilatation. Intraductal hyperplasia is seen and is generally of similar appearance to that seen in the female (Plate P.6.10). The male breast does not contain TDLUs but there are occasional reports of some degree of lobular development in gynaecomastia, particularly in patients with prostatic carcinoma on long-term stilboestrol therapy. The stroma is cellular, vascular and often myxoid especially around the ducts. There may be an increase in lymphocytes and plasma cells.

In the inactive form, there is no perceptible increase in the number of ducts nor evidence of intraductal hyperplasia. The stroma is hyalinised and usually replaces the adipose tissue. The periductal stroma shows no special features. About one third of cases show an appearance intermediate between the active and inactive forms.

These different histological appearances relate to the duration of the condition rather than its aetiology.

Table 6.5   Causes of gynaecomastia
Physiological   Commonly occurs in the neonate, during puberty and in senescence

Reduced androgen production
    Congenital aplasia or hypoplasia of the testes
    Secondary testicular failure: following inflammation, trauma, surgery

Increased production of oestrogen   Neoplasm: testicular tumours, lung carcinomas, adrenal tumours
Increased peripheral aromatisation of androgen   Systemic disorders: liver dysfunction, chronic renal failure, chronic pulmonary disease, malnutrition

Drug-induced
    Oestrogenic activity — oestrogen, digitalis
    Antiandrogenic properties — cyproterone, cimetidine, spironolactone
    Disturbance of gonadotropin control — phenothiazines, reserpine, methyldopa
    Germinal epithelial damage — cytotoxic drugs

Idiopathic

ULTRASONIC FEATURES

Two ultrasonic patterns are recognised[30]:

1. An echo-poor mass in the retroareolar area (Fig. 6.29). The mass is usually oval or triangular in shape and well-circumscribed. The appearance is similar to the pubertal breast (see Ch. 2.5), the histology being identical. This type corresponds with the active form and must be distinguished from male breast carcinoma, significant characteristics being the absence of invasive features (e.g. a halo), calcification or skin thickening.

2. A diffuse echogenic area in the breast (Fig. 6.30). The texture is similar to that of the normal glandular parenchyma of the mature female breast. This type correlates with the inactive (fibrous) type histologically.

Fig. 6.29
Gynaecomastia (echo-poor type)
This man presented with a unilateral breast lump. On ultrasound an oval, well-circumscribed echo-poor nodule is seen in the subareolar region. Histologically this was an active phase (florid type) gynaecomastia.

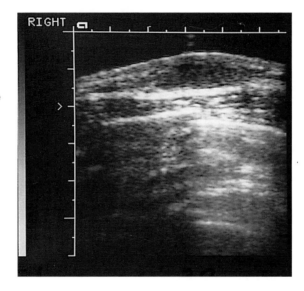

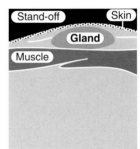

REFERENCES

24. N. Treves: Gynecomastia. The origins of mammary swelling in the male: an analysis of 406 patients with breast hypertrophy, 525 with testicular tumors, and 13 with adrenal neoplasms. Cancer 11; 1082–1102, 1958.
25. C.C. Kapdi, N.J. Parekh: The male breast. Radiol Clin North Am 21; 137–148, 1983.
26. L.E. Hughes, R.E. Mansel, D.V.T. Webster: Benign Disorders and Diseases of the Breast. Baillière Tindall, London, 1989, pp 167–172.
27. M.J. Williams: Gynecomastia: its incidence, recognition and host characterization in 447 autopsy cases. Am J Med 34; 103–112, 1963.
28. J.A. Andersen, J.B. Gram: Gynecomasty: histological aspects in a surgical material. Acta Pathol Microbiol Immunol Scand 90; 185–190, 1982.
29. G.A. Bannayan, S.I. Hajdu: Gynecomastia: clinicopathologic study of 351 cases. Am J Clin Pathol 57; 431–437, 1972.
30. K.D. Wigley, J.L. Thomas, M.E. Bernardino, J.L. Rosenbaum: Sonography of gynecomastia. AJR 136; 927–930, 1981.

Fig. 6.30
Gynaecomastia (echogenic type)

a. This man had a CT scan for evaluation of a carcinoid tumour of the lung. A soft tissue mass was found in the left breast. On ultrasound, an echogenic glandular tissue with ductal structures is seen in the retroareolar region.

b. Scan of the opposite breast which did not contain glandular components.

c. Following chemotherapy for Hodgkin's disease, this man noticed breast swelling. The echogenic glandular tissue is very similar to that in a female breast.

SCF: subcutaneous fat

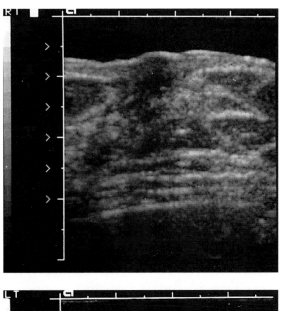
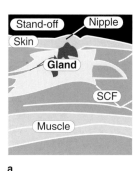

a

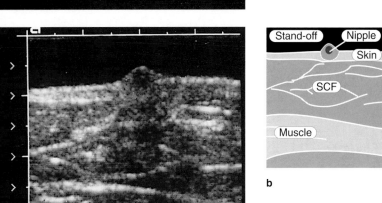

b

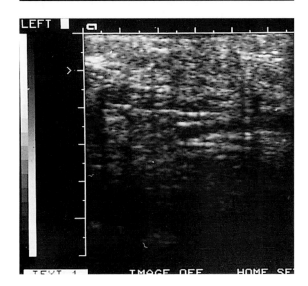
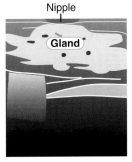

c

Chapter 7

Benign processes – inflammation

CLINICAL FEATURES

Commonly known as 'mastitis', breast inflammation is distinct from the type of benign breast change sometimes termed 'chronic mastitis'. Since benign breast change may also cause pain, this confusion is understandably common among patients. Benign breast change is neither infective nor usually inflammatory, while duct ectasia may be classified under either benign breast change or inflammation. Inflammation of the breast can be divided into infectious and non-infectious types (Table 7.1).

The organisms responsible for infectious mastitis are the common pyogenic bacteria such as *Staphylococcus aureus*; other organisms are very rare, especially in developed countries.

Lactational mastitis is the commonest true inflammatory disease of the breast. A cracked nipple during lactation allows bacteria to gain entry and at the same time occludes the duct orifices. Stasis of milk provides the ideal conditions for bacterial proliferation resulting in pain, redness and a hot breast. This common puerperal complication is easily diagnosed clinically.

Subareolar abscesses tend to recur in women with an inverted nipple. Squamous metaplasia of the nipple duct is considered to be a contributing factor because the orifice becomes plugged by keratin debris. Fistula formation to the skin may follow the recurrent infections. Simple drainage of the abscess is usually inadequate, complete excision of the affected duct being required to prevent recurrence. This is usually deferred until the acute phase has responded to antibiotics.

Other non-specific types of inflammation may occur in middle-aged women, probably due to retrograde infection along dilated ducts; occasionally also cysts become infected. These cases must be differentiated from inflammatory carcinomas, the most serious type of breast carcinoma. True inflammation tends to be more localised than an inflammatory carcinoma and is usually accompanied by leucocytosis and fever. It also responds quickly to antibiotic treatment; if the inflammation does not disappear completely after such treatment, skin biopsy is required to rule out an inflammatory carcinoma.

Sebaceous cysts or Montgomery's glands (sebaceous glands in the areola) may become secondarily infected. The appearance of a sebaceous cyst is described in Chapter 6.1.

Duct ectasia, also known as 'plasma cell mastitis' or 'periductal mastitis', is important because of its similarity to malignancy both clinically and on mammography[1–3]. The ducts become distended with secretions which may be discharged onto the nipple where it may occasionally induce eczematous changes that resemble Paget's disease. Sometimes the discharge is blood-stained. The ducts are often palpable and are described as a 'doughy, worm-like mass'. Aseptic inflammation occurs in response to the chemical irritation caused by the materials in the duct leaking through ulcerated ductal epithelium. The associated inflammation and fibrosis may lead to nipple retraction or a hard mass, either of which is suspicious of carcinoma. Diagnostic clues are the typical subareolar location, the bilaterality of the nipple retraction and the discharge. The course is usually chronic but may be acute, with evolution over a few days and rapid resolution or

Table 7.1	Inflammation of the breast	
	Factors	Special category
Infectious	Lactation	Lactational mastitis
	Inverted nipple	Subareolar abscess
	Non-specific	Dilated duct or cyst
	Sebaceous cyst	
	Montgomery's gland	
Non-infectious	Duct dilatation	Duct ectasia
	Trauma	Fat necrosis
	Malignancy	Inflammatory carcinoma

gradual progression to nipple retraction. The acute phase seems to be precipitated by rupture of the ducts. Duct ectasia may cause linear calcifications on the mammogram.

Fat necrosis is often included in the category of inflammation, here a chemical irritation by released lipids. It is described in Chapter 8.1. Inflammatory carcinoma is described in Chapter 9.5.

PATHOLOGICAL FEATURES

Acute pyogenic infections exhibit the same pathological features of acute inflammation, with or without abscess formation, as elsewhere.

The condition of recurring subareolar abscess (mammary duct fistula) is characterised by an eccentric subareolar lump which periodically discharges onto the areola. Histological examination reveals a fistulous tract extending from the surface of the areola to a main subareolar mammary duct which exhibits squamous metaplasia and is occluded by debris and cornified epithelial cells (Plate P.7.1). It is not known whether the squamous metaplasia is secondary to the inflammation or the cause of it.

Major duct ectasia (Plate P.7.2) involves mainly the large subareolar ducts although the process may extend into the smaller ones. The ducts are distended by thick white or green material which is deeply eosinophilic in histological sections. There is usually marked periductal infiltration by lymphocytes, plasma cells and histiocytes together with a significant degree of periductal fibrosis. The terms 'periductal mastitis' and 'plasma cell mastitis' are often applied in view of the inflammation, although the plasma cell component is rarely dominant. Many foamy histiocytes are often present, usually within the lumen but also in the periductal tissues. The periductal fibrosis is not always concentric and may take the form of irregular plaques that produce marked ductal distortion. Sometimes the process leads to complete ductal obliteration.

ULTRASOUND FEATURES

Infection

Inflammation due to bacterial infection initially produces a cellulitis with skin thickening and a diffuse increase in the subcutaneous fat echoes (Fig. 7.1). The glandular tissue is also thickened and the interface between the gland and the subcutaneous fat is blurred. Slight shadowing may be seen. The appearances are similar to those of inflammatory breast carcinoma, but less extensive.

In the second phase, the inflammatory exudate and white blood cells collect to form an abscess (Fig. 7.2). An abscess usually has irregular walls with a heterogeneous cavity comprising a mixture of cystic and solid portions. The posterior echoes are usually enhanced because of the fluid it contains. The hyperaemia is well shown on a colour Doppler examination which reveals many vessels with high velocity blood flow in the wall and around the lesion but not in its fluid centre (Plate C.12). An abscess cavity usually needs to be drained and this can often be expedited by using ultrasound guidance.

Fig. 7.1
Mastitis (cellulitis phase)
This 51-year-old lady developed marked breast tenderness. On ultrasound, thickening of the skin (★) and glandular tissue, a slight increase in the echogenicity of the subcutaneous fat (★★) and shadowing from the thick glandular tissue were observed. The symptoms disappeared completely after treatment with antibiotics.

RMS: retromammary space
SCF: subcutaneous fat

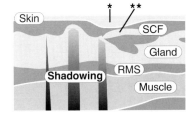

Fig. 7.2
Breast abscesses
a. This patient, who was receiving corticosteroids for systemic lupus erythematosus, suddenly developed a painful breast mass. The cystic lesion with irregular solid components has the typical ultrasound appearance of a breast abscess. The skin is thickened but, because of the reduced echogenicity of the oedematous skin and the increased echogenicity of the inflamed subcutaneous fat, the skin/fat interface is blurred.
b. One week after a fine needle aspiration for cytology (the result was benign: C2), the breast in this patient became swollen and reddened. On ultrasound, a thick walled cavity with some echogenic portions and distal enhancement is seen. This abscess was drained surgically.

GI: mammary gland
PE: posterior enhancement

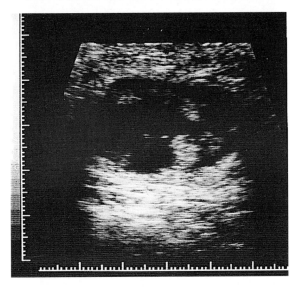

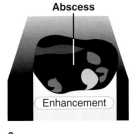

a

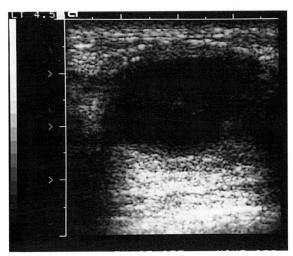

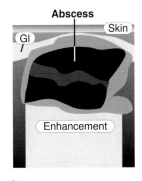

b

Rare infectious diseases

Though tuberculosis in general is common, it rarely involves the breast. Two types are recognised: primary and secondary. In primary cases the breast is the only site of infection, the organism having gained entry through the duct system. Secondary involvement is haematogenous or lymphatic. Breast lesions may be seen as circumscribed nodules, nodules with fibrosis, which are clinically similar to carcinomas, or as ulcers[4,5]. No specific ultrasound features have been reported.

Underlying pleural tuberculosis may penetrate through the chest wall directly and form a breast mass; in fact this is a cold abscess. Ultrasound is useful for demonstrating the 'collar stud' continuity between the mass and the pleural cavity, while movement of the contents between the two spaces can be observed during gentle pressure on the cavity, thus confirming its fluid content.

Blastmycosis is reported to form solid nodules which may cavitate with a resulting air–fluid level[6].

Subareolar abscess

The features of subareolar abscesses are similar to abscess forming in the parenchyma, as already described. An echo-poor region is seen under the nipple. The reaction may be more subtle than in acute infection.

Duct ectasia

Duct dilatation is a very common finding on ultrasound and, if asymptomatic, is considered as part of benign breast change. The typical ultrasound appearance is a dilated duct in the subareolar region which may not be entirely echo-free because it contains cellular debris or lipids (Fig. 7.3). Periductal inflammation may be seen as thickening of the duct wall or as an ill-defined border to the duct.

Fig. 7.3
Duct ectasia
This 60-year-old woman presented with gradually increasing retraction of the right nipple associated with a hard mass. A markedly dilated duct with weak internal echoes is seen. Fine needle aspiration retrieved inflammatory and foam cells which are typical of duct ectasia. Usually the contents of the ducts are more echogenic and the duct wall thickening is more prominent.

ES: edge shadow
GI: mammary gland
SCF: subcutaneous fat

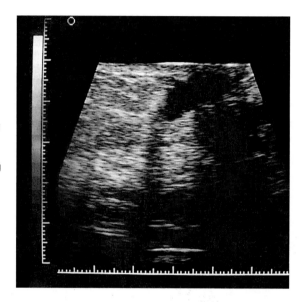

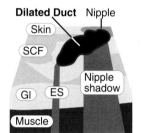

REFERENCES

1. J.C. Bloodgood: The clinical picture of dilated ducts beneath the nipple frequently to be palpated as a doughy worm-like mass — the varicocele tumor of the breast. Surg Gynecol Obstet 36; 486–495, 1923.
2. C.D. Haagensen: Mammary duct ectasia; a disease that may simulate carcinoma. Cancer 4; 749–761, 1951.
3. M. Ewing: Stagnation in the main ducts of the breast. J R Coll Surg Edinb 8; 134–144, 1963.
4. R.W. Raven: Tuberculosis of the breast. BMJ ; 734–736, 1949.
5. J.A. Hale, G.N. Peters, J.H. Cheek: Tuberculosis of the breast: rare but still extant. Am J Surg 50; 620–624, 1985.
6. E.O. Seymour: Blastomycosis of the breast. AJR 139; 822–823, 1982.

Chapter 8

Benign processes – trauma and iatrogenic conditions

8.1 FAT NECROSIS

CLINICAL FEATURES

Fat necrosis most often occurs in fatty, pendulous breasts. Though it is presumed to be traumatic in origin, a history of injury is only forthcoming in 40% of patients[1]. The condition is not always clinically manifest, the typical mammographic appearances of a radiolucent round lesion with a calcified wall often being an incidental finding[2]. Fat necrosis may also follow surgical trauma, especially at the site of a wide local excision for carcinoma followed by radiotherapy[3]; postradiation endarteritis obliterans with subsequent ischaemia has been suggested as a possible cause. In these cases the important differential diagnosis is from local recurrence of the tumour. Fat necrosis may also follow rupture of cysts or of ectatic ducts.

There are two forms of fat necrosis, depending on the reaction of the surrounding breast and they differ clinically, mammographically and ultrasonographically. When the fat necrosis stimulates a fibrotic response, it presents as a firm mass that is fixed to the surrounding tissues. It may also cause retraction of the skin or nipple, thus mimicking a carcinoma. The other type forms an oil cyst due to release of free lipid without eliciting a surrounding reaction. A rounded, well-delineated mass is palpable. The mammographic appearance of an oil cyst is a very characteristic thin walled nodule with a radiolucent centre[4,5].

PATHOLOGICAL FEATURES

Traumatic necrosis of the adipose tissue leads to breaking-up of the adipocytes from which fat is liberated and taken up by macrophages which thus acquire copious vacuolated cytoplasm. Lipid-filled spaces and lipid crystals may also be seen. The necrotic tissue and free lipid become surrounded by a foreign body type giant cell granulomatous reaction which proceeds to fibrosis. Deposits of haemosiderin are observed. In the later phases of the process the lesion becomes progressively more fibrotic, producing a hard irregular mass which may be mistaken for a carcinoma on macroscopic examination (Plate P.8.1).

ULTRASOUND FEATURES

Fat necrosis surrounded by a fibrous reaction has an identical ultrasonic appearance to a scirrhous breast carcinoma and is as confusing on ultrasound as on palpation and mammography. Postoperative scars do not usually have a nidus but, if accompanied by fat necrosis, they may have an echo-poor central nidus consisting of fibrous tissue that has replaced the necrotic fat. The surrounding abundant fibrosis causes an irregular and invasive appearance with posterior shadowing (Fig. 8.1), all of which are also features typical of a carcinoma.

Fig. 8.1
Fat necrosis

a. 6 years after lumpectomy and radiotherapy for an infiltrating ductal carcinoma, a 1.2 cm firm lump was felt at the site of the scar. The irregular-shaped shadowing lesion with a halo is very suspicious on ultrasound and tumour recurrence was suspected. However, on histology fibrosis with no malignancy was found.

b. This lesion was found when ultrasound was performed for radiotherapy planning after wide local excision. The appearance was considered suspicious of local recurrence or residual tumour but did not change during a year's follow-up.

c. 1 year after a wide local excision for an invasive carcinoma, this patient developed a tender nodule at the site of the scar. Because of the echo-poor nidus in the echogenic fibrous tissue, tumour recurrence was suspected. Histologically only fat necrosis was present.

RMS: retromammary space
SCF: subcutaneous fat

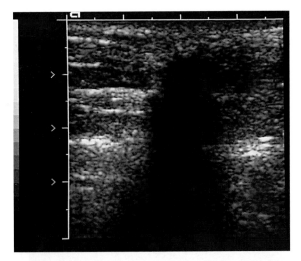

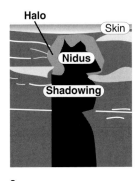

a

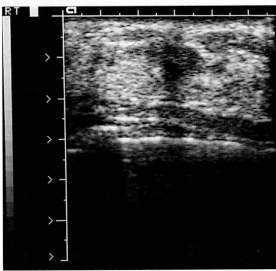

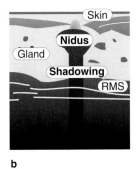

b

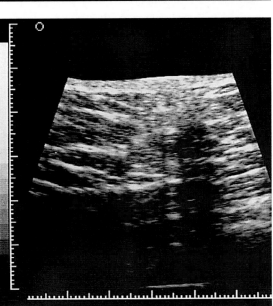

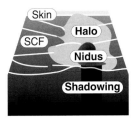

c

Fig. 8.2
Postoperative oil cyst

a. A well-circumscribed echo-poor area with slight shadowing was seen under the scar 1 year after excision of an infiltrating ductal carcinoma. The lesion was removed on suspicion of recurrent tumour but histology showed a cyst with fat necrosis, fibrosis, chronic inflammation and foreign body giant cells in the wall.

b. This woman had a biopsy for benign disease 1 year previously. A nodule was palpable medial to the scar. On ultrasound, a well-defined echogenic mass with posterior shadowing is seen. The high level echoes would be very unusual in breast tumours, which are almost always echo-poor — granuloma was the suggested diagnosis. On mammography the diagnosis was obvious: a well-encapsulated radiolucent mass, typical of an oil cyst was found (**c**).

ES: edge shadow
GI: mammary gland
SCF: subcutaneous fat

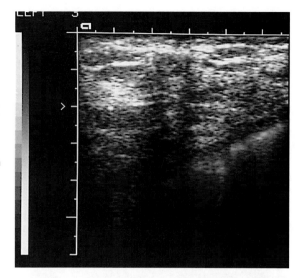

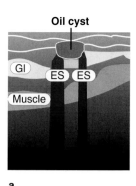

a

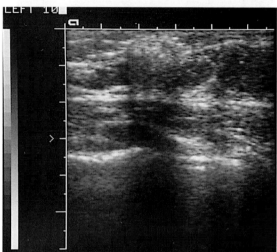

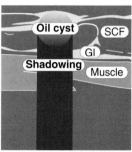

b

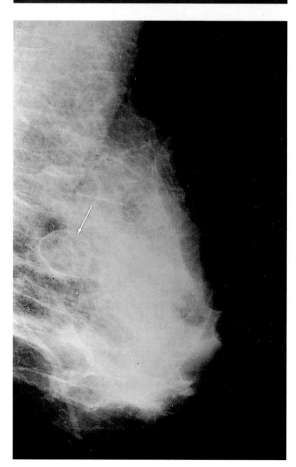

c

Oil cysts have a variety of appearances. They may be seen as simple cysts[4], or may resemble solid lesions because of the internal echoes and posterior attenuation (Fig. 8.2). A pathognomonic feature is the formation of a fluid level between the supernatant lipid, which is echogenic, and the denser watery component, which is anechoic (see Ch. 2, Fig. 2.13). This pattern is the reverse of the fluid–fluid level in haemorrhagic cysts (see Ch. 4, Fig. 4.13). When the lipid component is small, the echogenic portion is easily misinterpreted as reverberation artefact. The demonstration of repositioning of the horizontal interface when the patient's position is changed is very useful in confirming the diagnosis. Oil cysts with calcified walls are seen as curvilinear strong echoes with shadowing (Fig. 8.3). They cannot be differentiated from simple cysts with calcified walls or from heavily calcified fibroadenomas because evaluation of internal echoes is precluded by the intense shadowing. Calcified fibroadenomas tend to have a slightly irregular border because the calcification usually occurs not at the surface but within the periphery of the lesion. The differentiation between calcified oil cysts, water-filled cysts and fibroadenomas may be made on mammography but is unimportant clinically because all are benign.

Fig. 8.3
Calcified oil cyst
This non-palpable breast lesion is seen as an intensely reflective ring shape with shadowing (**a**). The appearance is typical of a calcified cyst. Evaluation of its internal echoes is precluded by the shadowing. A radiolucent centre on the mammogram confirmed it to be an oil cyst (**b**).

SCF: subcutaneous fat

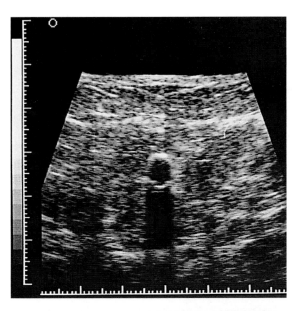
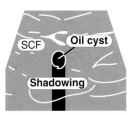

a

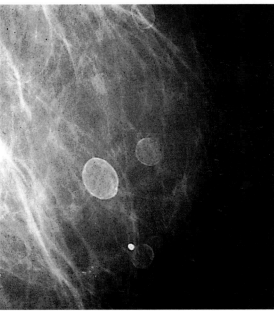

b

REFERENCES

1. C.D. Haagensen: Disease of the Breast (3rd edn). W.B. Saunders, Philadelphia, 1986, pp 369–378.
2. L.W. Orson, O.S. Cigtay: Fat necrosis of the breast: characteristic xeromammographic appearance. Radiology 146; 35–38, 1983.
3. A.Y. Rostom, M.E. El-Sayed: Fat necrosis of the breast: an unusual complication of lumpectomy and radiotherapy in breast cancer. Clini Radiology 38; 31, 1987.
4. C.L. Morgan, W.S. Trought, W. Peete: Xeromammographic and ultrasonic diagnosis of a traumatic oil cyst. AJR 130; 1189–1190, 1978.
5. L.W. Bassett, R.H. Gold, H.C. Cove: Mammographic spectrum of traumatic fat necrosis: the fallibility of 'pathognomonic' signs of carcinoma. AJR 130; 119–122, 1978.

8.2 HAEMATOMA

CLINICAL FEATURES

Haematoma occurs after trauma, either accidental or iatrogenic. Spontaneous bleeding into the breast is rare and requires investigation for an underlying cause, of which the most important is an occult carcinoma.

Haematomas are usually accompanied by bruising of the skin. Large haematomas are often complications of excisional biopsy because blood accumulates in the dead space. They may not be recognised clinically, many unsuspected postoperative cavities being demonstrable on ultrasound.

ULTRASOUND FEATURES

Haematomas are collections of blood but the distribution of the blood and the state of coagulation determine the precise ultrasound appearance. The cavity may be anechoic (Fig. 8.4.a) or contain low level (Fig. 8.4.b, c) or even strong internal echoes (Fig. 8.4.d), depending on the degree of organisation of the blood[6,7]. Inflammatory changes in the tissue around the haematoma may form an echogenic area around the cavity. Bleeding with haematoma formation occasionally occurs even after fine needle aspiration (Fig. 8.5).

Fig. 8.4
Haematomas
a. A breast lump developed after a dog bite 4 weeks before the scan. The lesion is almost anechoic, accompanied by posterior enhancement, an appearance that is similar to a simple cyst. However, an echogenic band around the fluid, due to an inflammatory reaction, suggests a traumatic origin. The overlying skin (★) is thickened and echo-poor because of oedema.
b. Following a severe chest injury, a wide area of bruising appeared on the breast in this patient. On ultrasound a large fluid collection is seen, with fine strands due to fibrin.

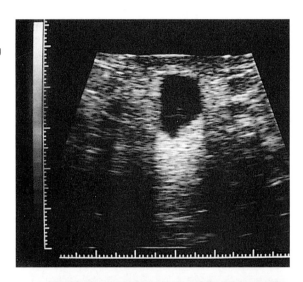
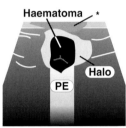

a

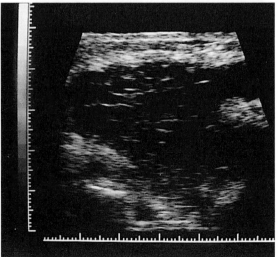
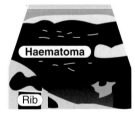

b

REFERENCES

6. G. Wolf, G. Hohenberg: Mammographic and sonographic appearances of traumatic changes in the female breast. ROFO 141; 204–208, 1984.

7. B. Gollentz, P. Ballarini, S. Rossier, D. Chague: Breast hematoma and cytosteatonecrosis. J Radiol 71; 33–43, 1990.

c. This ultrasound examination was performed 18 days after excision biopsy for an intraductal carcinoma found on screening mammography. The fibrin meshwork in the haematoma forms thicker and more obvious strands than in (**b**).

d. This haematoma was scanned 18 months after wide local excision for an invasive carcinoma. It has become organised and is almost solid.

ES: edge shadow
PE: posterior enhancement

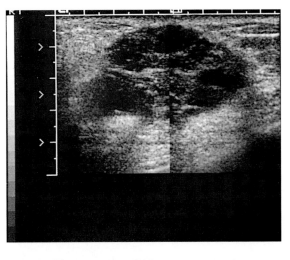
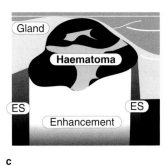

c

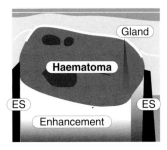

d

Fig. 8.5
Bleeding after fine needle aspiration cytology (FNAC)

a. A faint ill-defined echogenic area is seen in the subcutaneous fat at the site of FNAC taken about 1 h before the scan. The lesion was not seen on the previous ultrasound and had disappeared a week later.

b. This woman had a FNAC for a breast carcinoma deep to this area 5 days previously (the carcinoma is not seen on this scan). An ill-defined echogenic area with fluid at its centre is seen in the subcutaneous fat. FNAC occasionally causes a haematoma with a very confusing appearance because the reaction to the bleeding is similar to the invasive margin around a carcinoma.

GI: mammary gland
SCF: subcutaneous fat

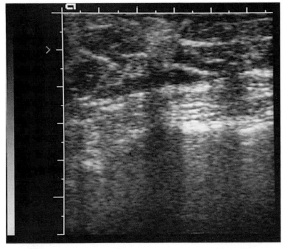
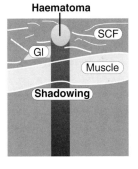

a

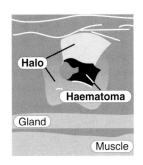

b

CLINICAL FEATURES

Scars in the breast usually do not pose a diagnostic problem unless accompanied by fat necrosis or when a locally recurring tumour is suspected, though occasionally tenderness interferes with palpation. There may be a palpable defect at the site of excision, making the cut edges of the breast tissue much more obvious than the scar itself. The position of postoperative scars can usually be anticipated from the history and by the skin incision site though, when the incision is circumareolar (as is usually performed for benign biopsies), the site of tissue removal may be some way from the skin scar.

ULTRASOUND FEATURES

Early changes following excision biopsy include inflammation (e.g. skin thickening and increased reflectivity of the subcutaneous fatty tissue) and distortion of the breast, including the formation of haematomas (Fig. 8.6). Ultrasound is rarely indicated during this phase except for the assessment of the size of the collection which usually resorbs gradually, though recovery time may be delayed by postoperative irradiation, which may also produce additional features (see Ch. 8.5).

In the later, stable phase, many scars, especially those following biopsies for benign diseases (for which only a small amount of tissue was excised), are completely invisible on ultrasound, a slight loss of breast tissue being the only change[8].

A narrow shadow is the commonest ultrasound finding in scarring (Fig. 8.7); it can be demonstrated in some 14% patients following lumpectomy and irradiation for breast carcinoma. The shadow may emanate from the skin, the subcutaneous tissues or from the glandular layer itself. The main cause of the shadow is probably stromal or textural distortion, though fibrosis also contributes[9]. This shadow may be broad if scanned along the length of the scar but is narrow when scanned across it. This characteristic three-dimensional configuration is an important sign in differentiating scar shadowing from that due to a tumour and is readily appreciated on real-time. Difficulties in retaining contact with the deformed skin also cause shadowing which is easily appreciated and compensated for with a hand-held real-time transducer. Similarly, the intense shadowing that may arise from the skin scar and interfere with visualisation of the underlying tissue may be avoided by scanning with the probe tilted to gain access from alongside the scar.

Scars usually do not have the echo-poor nidus that is suggestive of recurrent tumour though fat necrosis and granulomas may produce a nidus. The differentiation between a scar and recurrent tumour is sometimes very difficult, though a rounded nodule or focal thickening of the 'scar' is suspicious (Fig. 8.8). Dynamic tests are not very helpful because, like carcinomas, scars are fixed to the surrounding tissue. They may be compressible but are often hard. Since a scar is avascular, the demonstration of blood vessels on colour Doppler is very suspicious of an underlying malignancy. Fine needle aspiration cytology is usually required and may usefully be guided by ultrasound to ensure that the suspicious region is sampled. Periodical follow-up ultrasound examinations are also helpful where a recurrence is suspected: any enlargement of the suspicious region warrants biopsy.

Fig. 8.6
Early changes in scarring
5 days after excisional biopsy, the breast is diffusely echogenic due to inflammatory change—the fatty tissue is particularly affected. The skin is thickened and the interface between the skin and the subcutaneous fat is obliterated. There is also a small haematoma .

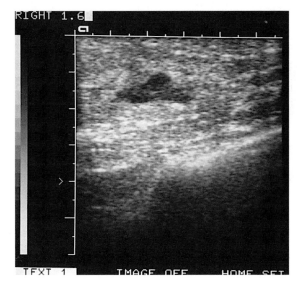
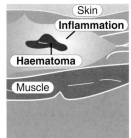

Fig. 8.7
Typical scars
Narrow shadows with slight distortion
of the breast texture but without an
echo-poor nidus are the typical
appearance of scars (**a**, **b**). Skin
thickening due to radiotherapy is also
seen in (**a**).

Gl: mammary gland
IS: interface shadow from a Cooper's
ligament
SCF: subcutaneous fat

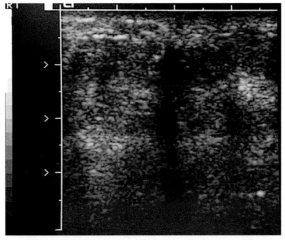
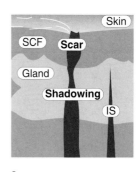

a

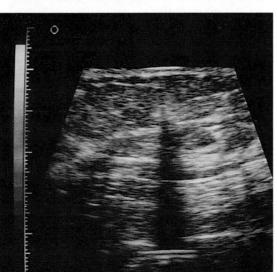
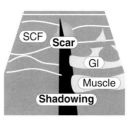

b

Fig. 8.8
Scar mimicking a breast carcinoma
A small echo-poor area in the breast
parenchyma mimics a tumour nidus
while echogenic fibrosis around it is
suggestive of a halo; the suspicion of
malignancy was heightened by the
shadowing. The 'mass' was excised
for histology but no tumour was found.

Gl: mammary gland
SCF: subcutaneous fat

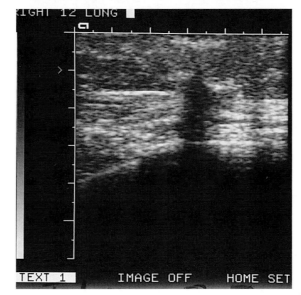
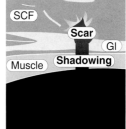

REFERENCES

8. W.J. Leucht, D.R. Rabe: Sonographic findings following conservative surgery and irradiation for breast carcinoma. Ultrasound Med
Biol 14 (suppl 1); 27–41, 1988.

9. G. Kossoff: Causes of shadowing in breast sonography. Ultrasound
Med Biol 14 (suppl 1); 211–215, 1988.

8.4 MAMMOPLASTY AND BREAST RECONSTRUCTION

CLINICAL FEATURES

Mammoplasty may be performed for augmentation or reduction of the breast. Reduction mammoplasty produces scars but usually does not cause special diagnostic problems apart from residual nodularity which may be felt in the central and lower parts of the breast, corresponding to the vertical limb of the scar.

Augmentation mammoplasty and breast reconstruction are usually performed using silicone prostheses. Injection of free silicone or paraffin into the breasts was used in the past but has been abandoned because of its hazards such as granuloma formation or migration of the implant material. Silicone bags are now usually used as prostheses because they are less likely to provoke a granulomatous reaction. They may be filled with silicone gel or saline. Saline can be injected after operation in the latter type to adjust the size of the prosthesis and prevent capsular fibrosis. For this, the prostheses are fitted with a filling port which is usually palpable but, if not, can readily be localised with ultrasound to expedite filling. In the tissue expansion technique, the temporary saline prosthesis

is inflated after operation to stretch the chest wall and skin and is subsequently replaced by a permanent implant filled with silicone at a second operation[10]. The Becker prosthesis with a double lumen comprising an outer bag filled with silicone gel (for shape and texture) and an inner lumen for saline (which can be filled later) has been introduced to avoid two operations[11].

The prostheses are usually inserted deep to the breast tissue, anterior to the pectoralis fascia or at the site of the defect after wide local excision. A method of insertion beneath the pectoralis muscle has been developed particularly for reconstruction after mastectomy to reduce the frequency of capsular contracture, which is one of the commonest complications affecting implants.

Early complications are haematoma and infection; these are usually obvious clinically and do not need confirmation by imaging. Late complications include deformity of the implant (due to leakage or rupture), capsular fibrosis, calcification and contraction.

Leakage or rupture of the bag may occur spontaneously but is more often caused by trauma. The implant

Fig. 8.9
Variations in the appearances of prostheses
a. Silicone prosthesis. Both silicone and saline prostheses are seen as an echo-free space. Reverberation artefacts usually affect the superficial portions, making the anterior wall seem thick.
b. Echoes may be seen within the prosthesis; they arise from wrinkles in the membrane, accentuated by side lobe and reverberation artefacts.

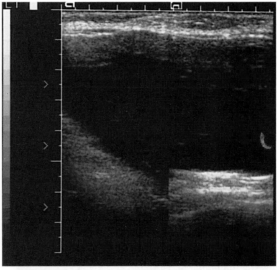

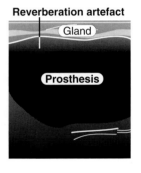

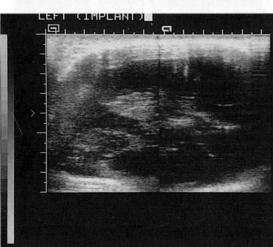

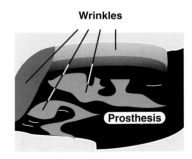

becomes deformed or forms palpable lumps but sometimes is asymptomatic.

Capsular fibrosis and contraction are clinically important because they make the reconstructed breast hard and uncomfortable or even painful. Closed capsulotomy (compressing the prosthesis manually to disrupt the capsule) often relieves the symptoms.

Silicone granulomas (Plate P.8.2) may be caused by small leakages of silicone gel, often after trauma or closed capsulotomy. Palpable lumps develop, usually located close to the prosthesis but sometimes affecting the regional lymph nodes. Asymptomatic granulomas are sometimes detected on ultrasound.

Any remaining breast is a potential site for disease, either benign or malignant. The glandular tissue is usually thin and superficially located and so is easily palpated. Mammography is of limited value because of the incompressibility of the breast and the density of the prosthesis. Fine needle aspiration cytology is better avoided because of the possibility of damage to the bag — when deemed necessary, it should be guided by ultrasound. Recurrent tumour is not a common problem because reconstruction is usually not indicated if the risk of recurrence is high but, if it occurs, it is difficult to diagnose and treat. This problem is discussed in Chapter 10.3.

Another technique for reconstruction employs a myo-cutaneous flap. The latissimus dorsi muscle is commonly used in combination with a silicone prosthesis. In the rectus abdominis myocutaneous flap reconstruction, the underlying subcutaneous fat may obviate the necessity for a prosthesis[10].

ULTRASOUND APPEARANCES

The appearances of the breast after reduction mammoplasty are the same as following excision biopsy (see Ch. 8.3). Attenuation and slight textural distortion of the breast tissue may be seen, but usually they do not cause special diagnostic problems.

The important applications of ultrasound are in augmented and reconstructed breasts[12]. Both saline and silicone prostheses are homogeneous materials and so are seen as anechoic spaces on ultrasound (Fig. 8.9.a). Reverberation artefacts between the skin and the prosthesis often affect the superficial part of the prosthesis while wrinkles in the membrane of the prosthesis may cause echoes of surprising shapes within the prosthesis (Fig. 8.9.b). Occasionally weak homogeneous internal echoes are seen in an old prosthesis, probably due to degeneration of the silicone (Fig. 8.9.c). Complicated reverberation artefacts are seen in double lumen prostheses (Fig. 8.9.d).

c. Homogeneous internal echoes in the prosthesis are true echoes, probably due to degeneration of the silicone.

d. Multiple lines are seen in the double lumen prosthesis (Becker's prosthesis). The filling port is also demonstrated — ultrasound is useful in localisation of the port for filling.

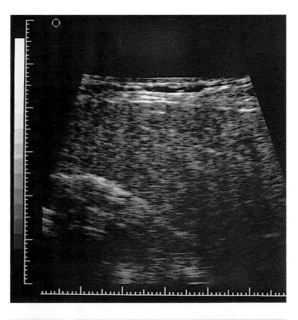

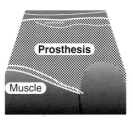

c

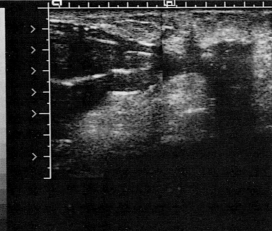

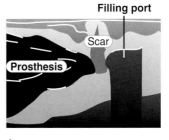

d

An interesting difference between silicone and saline prostheses is caused by the sound velocity in silicone being about half of that in normal breast tissue or saline; thus the scanner is incorrectly calibrated for depth in the silicone, causing the implant to be displayed as twice its real thickness (Fig. 8.10). Usually the posterior wall of the prosthesis is so deep as to lie beyond the limit of the image scale used for normal scanning for breasts. However, visualisation of deeper structures is not diagnostically important because usually there is no glandular tissue behind the implant.

Fig. 8.10
Velocity artefact
Because the sound velocity in the silicone implant is about half that in the glandular tissue of the breast, the prosthesis is depicted as twice as deep as its actual thickness — note the shelf-like displacement of the pleural layer.
This image was taken with a 3 MHz transducer to show the whole thickness of the prosthesis. Usually the posterior wall of the prosthesis is too deep to be seen on the image scale for breast scanning.

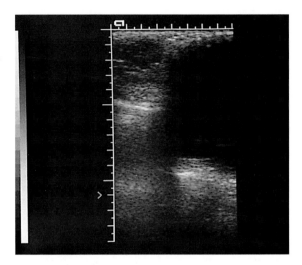

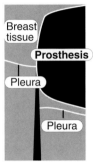

Deformity, rupture or leakage are seen as distortion of the prosthesis (Fig. 8.11) or as cystic spaces around the implant.

Ultrasound is usually not indicated to demonstrate capsular fibrosis or contraction because these are clinically obvious; the fibrosis produces bright parallel lines at the surfaces of the prosthesis[12].

Fig. 8.11
Deformity of an implant
This woman noticed a lump at the margin of the prosthesis. The edge of the prosthesis is deformed and expanded at the site of the palpable lump (**a**). The change is more obvious when compared with the unaffected part (★ in **b**).

RA: reverberation artefact

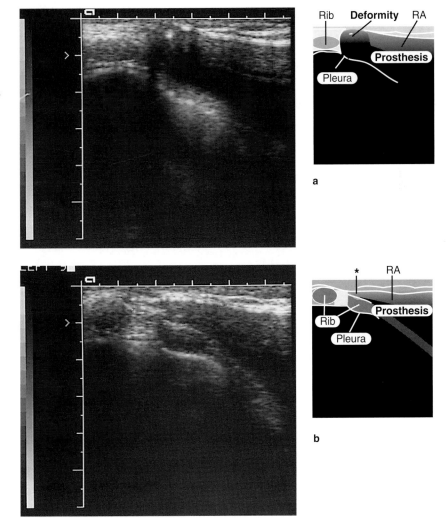

The ultrasound appearances of silicone granulomas are very characteristic. They are seen as relatively well-circumscribed echogenic masses with shadowing (Fig. 8.12)[13]. They may be extensive and the same features may develop in affected lymph nodes. Scattering is the cause of the high echogenicity and absorption is the cause of the attenuation. Curvilinear echogenic lines may be seen at the surface, due to the fibrous capsule. Echogenic masses are very rare in breast pathology, the only other causes being some fibrolipomas, oil cysts and calcification. Lipomas usually do not produce attenuation; calcification usually causes both very strong reflection and attenuation of ultrasound originating from the surface and it is seen as an echogenic line rather than as a mass.

Fig. 8.12
Silicone granulomas
a. This woman developed two lumps at the edge of the prosthesis in the right breast. She had had closed capsulotomies on both sides some 2 months earlier. Ultrasound revealed three masses, one of which was impalpable, all with similar appearances: well-circumscribed echogenic masses with posterior attenuation, typical of granulomas. The curvilinear intense echo at the surface of the mass is probably due to fibrosis. The palpable lumps were excised and proved to be silicone granulomas on histology.
b. 9 months later she found another lump in the opposite breast. The ultrasound appearances are very similar to those obtained previously (**a**).
c. Silicone granulomas may form at the surface of the prosthesis. This woman also has four similar lesions in both breasts, only one of which was palpable.

GI: mammary gland

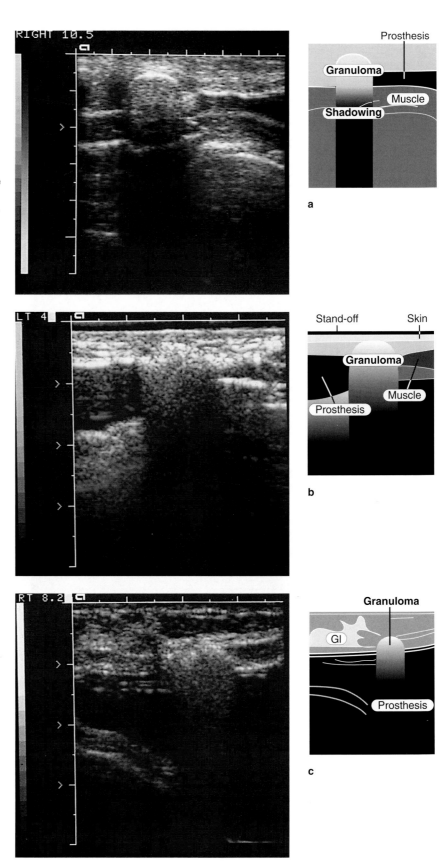

The presence of a breast implant does not reduce the effectiveness of ultrasound in the detection of parenchymal pathology as much as it does for mammography (Fig. 8.13). In augmented breasts, the thin glandular tissues are located at the surface of the breast or around the prosthesis, so that the focus of the ultrasound must be adjusted accordingly, but the ultrasound appearances of breast diseases are the same as those in breasts without implants. Dynamic tests are often difficult because of the stiffness of the prosthesis and the stretched skin.

Fig. 8.13
Breast carcinoma in an augmented breast
Any breast pathology may occur in the glandular parenchyma of an augmented breast. The prosthesis does not interfere with the visualisation of breast disease on ultrasound.

Ca: carcinoma
Gl: mammary gland
SL: superficial layer of the superficial fascia

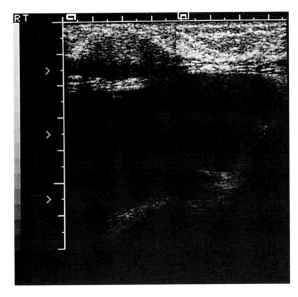
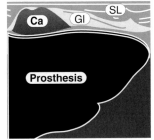

REFERENCES

1. W.D. McInnis: Plastic surgery of the breast. The Female Breast and Its Disorders, edited by G.W. Mitchell and L.W. Bassett. Williams & Wilkins, Baltimore, 1990, pp 196–217.
2. H. Becker: The permanent tissue expander. Clin Plast Surg 14; 519–527, 1987.
3. C. Cole-Beuglet, G. Schwartz, A.B. Kurtz, et al: Ultrasound mammography for the augmented breast. Radiology 146; 737–742, 1983.
4. P. Herzog: Silicone granulomas: detection by ultrasonography. Plast Reconstr Surg 84; 856–857, 1989.

8.5 IRRADIATED BREAST

CLINICAL FEATURES

Radiotherapy is commonly used for early breast carcinoma (stages I and II) in combination with conservative surgery. External irradiation after excision of the mass is the usual procedure, though interstitial radiotherapy, using iridium wires, has also been employed. Whole breast irradiation of moderate dose (40–60 Gy), sometimes with a boost for the region of the primary tumour, is standard treatment. The axillary region is not usually included if an axillary dissection has been performed.

Radiotherapy is also used as primary treatment, together with chemotherapy, for locally advanced carcinomas and especially for inflammatory carcinomas.

Clinical follow-up examination of the irradiated breast can be difficult because of skin thickening and induration.

PATHOLOGY

Histologically, the terminal duct lobular units may show degeneration and loss of epithelial cells usually with preservation of the myoepithelium. Some of the residual cells exhibit enlarged pleomorphic, hyperchromatic nuclei which can be mistaken for ductal carcinoma in situ if the history of irradiation is not known. These changes are generally followed by lobular atrophy and fibrosis (Plate P.8.3).

ULTRASOUND FEATURES

The changes which are commonly seen are[14–16]:

1. Skin thickening (Fig. 8.14)
2. Increased echogenicity in the subcutaneous fat (Fig. 8.15.a)
3. Thickening, distortion or blurring of the Cooper's ligaments (Fig. 8.15.b)
4. Architectural distortion of the breast tissue.

Some of these changes are due to the combined effects of radiotherapy and surgery, which usually also includes axillary dissection.

Thickening of the skin is the commonest change (60–95% of patients) and is best detected by comparison with the opposite breast (normal thickness <3 mm). The echogenicity of the skin is usually also increased in comparison with the opposite breast[16], though the increased echogenicity is most marked in the subcutaneous fat so that decreased contrast between the subcutaneous fat and the glandular tissue is one of the characteristic features of the irradiated breast. The featureless image that results is also seen in inflammation and in lymphoedema of the breast and is probably due to increased interstitial fluid. Thickening of Cooper's ligaments and distortion of breast texture may be due to surgery but fibrotic change and contraction may also be factors.

These changes are most often seen early after radiation; they usually last for a few months, gradually improving over the first year[15], but some abnormalities persist for several years[16]. Changes cannot always be demonstrated and the irradiated breast may have a completely normal appearance on ultrasound.

Ultrasound is mainly used in the irradiated breast to detect recurrent tumour or to assess a primary tumour treated by radiotherapy. The changes due to radiation usually do not affect the ability of ultrasound to detect a lesion, though focal scars are sometimes indistinguishable from recurrent tumour and decreased penetration of the sound beam occasionally makes visualisation of the deeper portions difficult. Recurrent carcinomas may have an unusual growth pattern, not forming a mass but spreading diffusely. This pattern is difficult to differentiate from the changes of irradiation.

Primary tumours become ill-defined following radiotherapy and may become undetectable as they regress.

REFERENCES

14. E.G. Grant, J.D. Richardson, O.S. Cigtay, et al: Sonography of the breast: findings following conservative surgery and irradiation for early carcinoma. Radiology 147; 535–539, 1983.
15. A.R. Calkins, V.P. Jackson, J.G. Morphis, F.B. Stehman: The sonographic appearance of the irradiated breast. J Clin Ultrasound 16; 409–415, 1988.
16. W.J. Leucht, D.R. Rabe: Sonographic findings following conservative surgery and irradiation for breast carcinoma. Ultrasound Med Biol 14 (suppl 1); 27–41, 1988.

Fig. 8.14
Thickening of the skin after irradiation
Three months after irradiation for a primary tumour the skin is slightly thickened and echogenic due to fibrosis. The interface between the glandular and fatty tissue layers is blurred and the normal layers of the skin are difficult to distinguish. The tumour is still detectable but is ill-defined.

Ca: carcinoma
SCF: subcutaneous fat

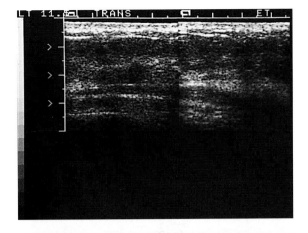
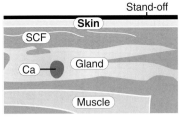

Fig. 8.15
Increased echogenicity of the subcutaneous fat after irradiation
This scan was taken some 6 weeks after completion of radiotherapy following excision of a carcinoma. Increased echogenicity of the subcutaneous tissue is more apparent (**a**) when compared with the opposite breast (**b**) (taken with the same gain settings). The contrast between the subcutaneous fat and the glandular tissue is reduced, giving the breast a featureless appearance.

RMS: retromammary space
SCF: subcutaneous fat
SL: superficial layer of the superficial fascia

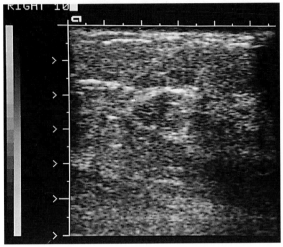
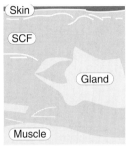

a

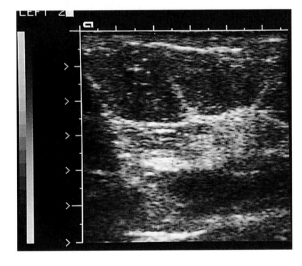
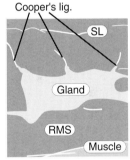

b

Chapter 9

Malignant disease – primary carcinomas

9.1 INVASIVE DUCTAL CARCINOMA

CLINICAL FEATURES

Invasive ductal carcinoma (also known as invasive carcinoma, no special type) is the commonest type of breast malignancy accounting for 70–80% of all breast carcinomas (Fig. 9.1)[1]. Because this is overwhelmingly the predominant malignancy, the general clinical and epidemiological aspects of breast cancer are discussed here.

The geographical incidence of breast carcinoma varies widely, being commoner in the West than in the East (Fig. 9.2)[2]. It is the commonest malignancy in women throughout almost all of Europe, North America and Australia, as well as in much of Latin America. The lifetime risk of developing breast carcinoma is 1 in 12 in the UK[3], with an incidence that rises progressively with age (Fig. 9.3)[4]. The incidence is particularly low in Japan but is much higher amongst Japanese immigrants to the USA, suggesting an environmental influence (e.g. diet) rather than or in addition to a genetic influence[5]. Both of these, as well as endocrine factors, have been suggested as aetiological or risk factors, although many remain controversial. Perhaps the best documented is the effect of oestrogens: in general, a high exposure to oestrogens predisposes to breast carcinoma. Typical factors are early onset of menstruation and late menopause[6], while there is an inverse relationship both with early age at first full-term birth and with the number of pregnancies[7], suggesting a protective effect of progesterones. The slightly increased incidence in younger women who have used oral contraceptives containing high dose oestrogens could be another manifestation of the same phenomenon, while progestogenic oral contraceptives are not thought to be linked with an increased risk[8]. The evidence that postmenopausal hormone replacement therapy (HRT) is associated with an increased risk is not conclusive[9].

Family history is a well-known risk factor, women with a first-degree relative (mother, sister or daughter) with a breast carcinoma having a two- to threefold likelihood of developing the disease[10,11]. In patients with a family history, the tumours tend to develop earlier (often before menopause) and are more likely to be bilateral[12].

The association between benign breast change and breast cancer is controversial. It now seems likely that only the hyperplastic components carry an increased risk

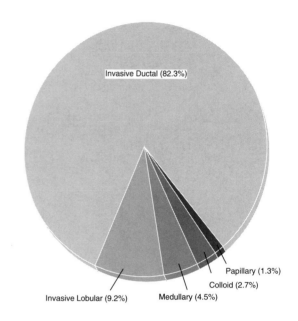

Fig. 9.1
Frequency of varieties of breast carcinoma
Invasive ductal carcinoma is the commonest type.

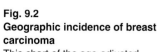

Fig. 9.2
Geographic incidence of breast carcinoma
This chart of the age-adjusted incidence of breast cancer by geographical area shows the high incidence in Western countries in contrast with the low incidence in the Far East.
[Redrawn from ref. 2.]

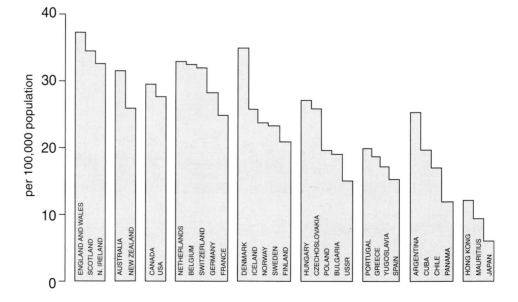

and this is most apparent if the hyperplasia is atypical and is associated with a family history of breast cancer (see Ch. 6.2).

The commonest presentation is with a lump in the breast, although generalised hardening or thickening may also occur. Most benign breast masses result from hormonal changes operating through the menstrual cycle and therefore typically enlarge toward the end of the cycle and regress after menstruation. By contrast, malignant masses enlarge progressively without cyclical changes. The appearance of a new mass after the menopause is particularly suspicious since the development of fibroadenomas or benign breast change is extremely unusual in this age group, except after stimulation by HRT.

Characteristically the mass of a breast carcinoma is solitary, hard, often irregular in contour and poorly delineated. The fixation within the breast tissues or to the pectoralis muscle that is typical of a carcinoma is extremely unusual in benign lesions. Pain is popularly considered to be reassuring but, in fact, occurs in about 15% of carcinomas and thus cannot be ignored as a presenting symptom. The pain is often described as 'pricking' in character.

Skin changes are important clinical signs of breast malignancy. Many carcinomas are surrounded by a fibrotic stromal reaction which shortens the Cooper's ligaments and the duct systems, producing flattening or dimpling of the overlying skin, together with flattening or even retraction of the nipple. Unilateral nipple retraction is a highly suspicious sign although bilateral retraction may occur in periductal mastitis, a disease of older women. Nipple retraction can be distinguished from congenital inversion of the nipples by the history (present since puberty) and bilaterality. Nipple discharge (see Ch. 5.3) occurs in only 10% but is particularly suspicious if it is blood-stained; most tumours presenting this way are minimally invasive or non-invasive. Neglected tumours may present with fungation. Skin oedema producing peau d'orange is discussed in the section on inflammatory carcinoma (see Ch. 9.5).

PATHOLOGICAL FEATURES

Invasive ductal carcinomas include all infiltrative carcinomas in the breast that lack special features and do not fall into any of the special subgroups. Consequently, they have a very variable appearance and may even show significant structural and cytological heterogeneity within the same lesion. Tumours which only partly exhibit features of any of the special subtypes are also included in this category. Despite the name, most of these tumours are now thought to arise from the terminal duct lobular units.

On macroscopic examination most are of the scirrhous type with an irregular stellate outline and a hard grey gritty cut surface, often with yellow flecks of elastin. Less commonly the tumours may be softer and circumscribed.

Histologically, the neoplastic cells usually grow in nests or cords but may form large masses. There is often a variable amount of tubule formation. Generally, the tumour cells are fairly uniform in size, shape and staining intensity but, in some tumours, there is marked pleomorphism.

Necrosis is not usually a prominent feature but may be seen in large and cellular tumours. Very rarely, densely cellular lesions may undergo extensive central necrosis.

The stroma is usually abundant and contains a large amount of collagen (Plate P.9.1) and, frequently, significant quantities of elastin. Microcalcification within the epithelium or stroma is a common feature; the calcific material is usually hydroxyapatite. The stroma also contains variable numbers of lymphocytes, plasma cells and histiocytes.

ULTRASOUND FEATURES

The majority (more than 90%) of infiltrating ductal carcinomas produce a mass on ultrasound imaging[13]. Therefore the ultrasonic features of the mass itself ('primary features') are the most important in detection and diagnosis, while the secondary features, relating to changes in the surrounding tissues, help confirm the malignant nature of the lesion but are more important in evaluating the degree of invasion. For lesions which do not produce a mass, only the secondary signs are available. In both groups dynamic and Doppler features are often also useful.

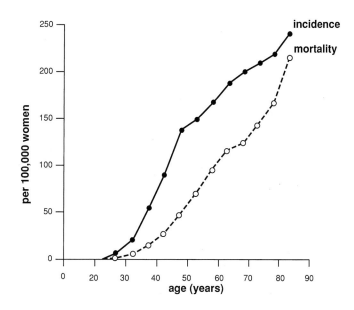

Fig. 9.3
Age specific incidence of breast cancer
The age specific incidence of breast cancer in the UK in 1982 shows the rapidly rising incidence with age as well as the typical flattening of the curve at menopause which is more clearly demonstrated on the mortality curve (UK for 1985). This feature lowers the overall totals somewhat. [Redrawn from ref. 4]

Primary features

The ultrasound features of breast carcinoma are very variable; heterogeneity of the lesion and signs of invasion are the most important. The mass itself is typically composed of two concentric layers (Fig. 9.4): a central nidus and an outer layer, known as the halo. The nidus is almost always less reflective than the surrounding glandular tissue and usually also less reflective than the subcutaneous fatty layer. Tumours that are highly calcified are a rare exception: they may be more reflective than breast parenchyma. The nidus usually has a heterogeneous texture (Fig. 9.5), perhaps due to the irregular alignment of the tumour cells or to patchy necrosis. In addition, microcalcification produces punctate echogenic foci which add to the heterogeneous texture (Fig. 9.6). Occasionally cystic change may be apparent (Fig. 9.7); it is more common with larger tumours and is probably due to necrosis or haemorrhage, this being supported by a typical location of the cystic region in the centre of the lesion (see Ch. 6.1 for intracystic tumours).

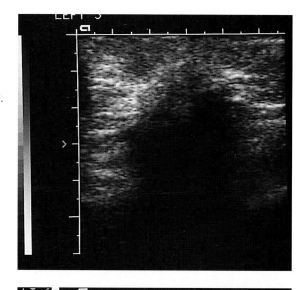
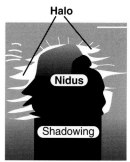

Fig. 9.4
Typical carcinoma
A mass of cancer cells and stromal tissues forms the echo-poor nidus. The invasive margin is seen as an echogenic zone around the nidus, termed the 'halo' or 'boundary echoes'. Shadowing is commonly seen, especially in tumours with a halo. Histologically these are usually scirrhous carcinomas.

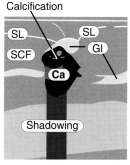

Fig. 9.5
Carcinoma with heterogeneous internal echoes
This carcinoma has heterogeneous internal echoes, party due to calcification. The shadowing and high D:W ratio are also typical features. The superficial tissues converge towards the tumour, a feature of malignancy that is caused by contraction of the fibrous tissues of the breast.

Ca: carcinoma
Gl: mammary gland
SCF: subcutaneous fat
SL: superficial layer of the superficial fascia

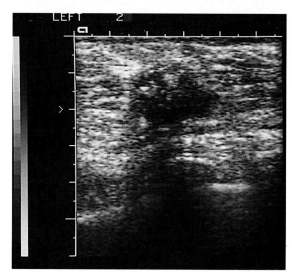
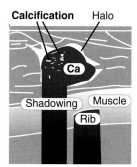

Fig. 9.6
Microcalcifications
a. Calcification in breast carcinomas usually takes the form of very small foci, seen as bright spots on ultrasound. Because they are smaller than the beam width, they do not cast an acoustic shadow, while the carcinoma itself often causes shadowing.

a

b. Mammogram of the same lesion.

Ca: carcinoma

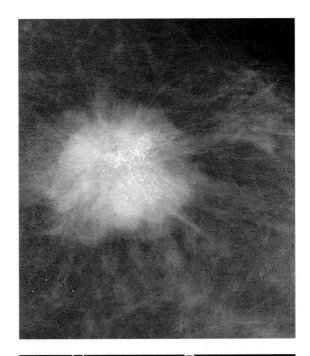

b

Fig. 9.7
Carcinoma with cystic change
a. This large lobulated tumour contains cystic spaces. The tumour itself is well-circumscribed and the posterior echoes are enhanced. The differential diagnosis on ultrasound was a phylloides tumour; histology of the excision biopsy showed a ductal carcinoma with haemorrhage. Cystic change due to haemorrhage or necrosis is sometimes seen in large tumours.

b. Rarely breast carcinomas present as a 'cyst'. The irregular structures within the cyst (★) and the slightly irregular wall (★★) are worrying appearances that make this lesion atypical of a simple cyst. Histologically, this was a highly necrotic tumour with an invasive ductal carcinoma in the wall.

ES: edge shadow
GI: mammary gland
SCF: subcutaneous fat
SL: superficial layer of the superficial fascia

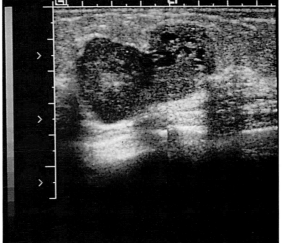

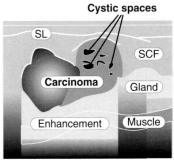

a

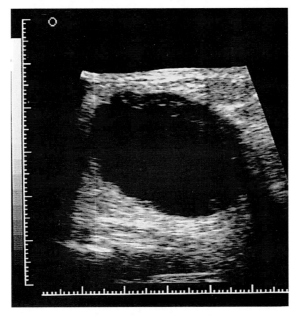

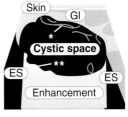

b

The tumour nidus is usually irregular in shape. A particular feature is the tendency of malignant lesions to grow anteriorly, crossing natural boundaries (Fig. 9.8). A tumour therefore tends to sit 'proud' in the breast, with its long axis lying anteroposteriorly. This is numerically evaluated as the depth:width (D:W) ratio which often exceeds 0.8 in breast carcinomas. This criterion is less useful with larger carcinomas; as these tend to be more irregular in shape, they are usually easily recognised even if they have a low D:W ratio.

The borders of invasive ductal carcinomas are irregular and usually appear ill-defined or fuzzy because of their invading margins (Fig. 9.9.a). This pattern is typical of the scirrhous type of tumour, while tumours with little desmoplastic reaction may have clear and well-defined margins, although they also are irregular or lobulated in shape (Fig. 9.9.b). The desmoplastic reaction around scirrhous tumours that causes the typical stellate appearance on mammograms is seen on ultrasound as an echogenic halo ('boundary echoes') around the lesion (Fig. 9.10.a), a feature that is almost specific of infiltrating breast carcinomas. (Rarely, non-malignant infiltrating processes, such as fat necrosis, have the same appearance.) The halo is more easily recognised against the background of an atrophic breast because of the high contrast with the echo-poor fat. It may be difficult to

detect within a glandular breast, especially on static images, because the halo has a similar echogenicity to the glandular tissue. In this situation dynamic tests (moving the lesion under the transducer) may clearly reveal the halo as an immobile zone attached to the nidus (Fig. 9.10.b). This sign is important in the differential diagnosis from fibroadenomas, especially those which show posterior shadowing; fibroadenomas never form an echogenic halo.

Fig. 9.8
Depth:width (D:W) ratio
a. This small tumour (8 mm) is almost round in shape and does not have a halo or heterogeneity of internal echoes. However, the high D:W ratio (1.0), posterior shadowing and the interruption of the adjacent structures are highly suspicious features. Cytology of the fine needle aspirate under ultrasound guidance was C4. Histology confirmed it to be an infiltrating ductal carcinoma.
b. This 3 cm tumour is flattened (low D:W ratio) but the irregular and fuzzy borders and posterior attenuation suggest a diagnosis of carcinoma. Large carcinomas tend to have lower D:W ratios.

GI: mammary gland
SL: superficial layer of the superficial fascia
SCF: subcutaneous fat

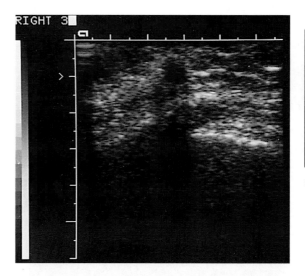

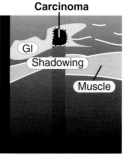

a

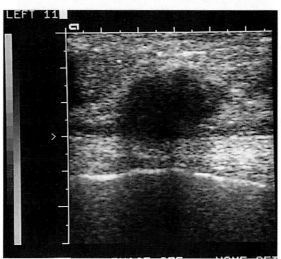

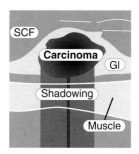

b

Fig. 9.9
Tumour margins
a. The irregular and ill-defined margins of this lesion suggest an invasive growth pattern. This is the typical appearance of an infiltrating carcinoma.
b. This lesion is well-circumscribed with a well-defined border and shows posterior echo enhancement. These are all benign features. However, the high D:W ratio and the lobulated margins are pointers to its malignant nature.

Gl: mammary gland
SCF: subcutaneous fat
Ca: carcinoma
RMS: tetromammary space

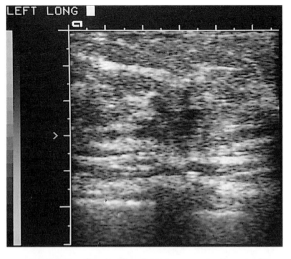
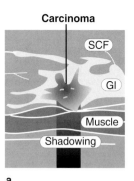

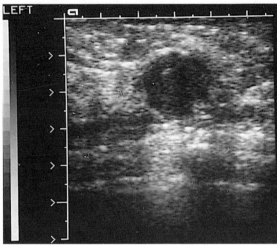
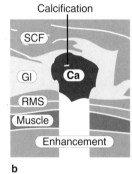

Fig. 9.10
Halo (boundary echoes)
a. This tumour with strong posterior attenuation has bright echoes around the echo-poor nidus. Known as a 'halo', they represent the infiltrating edge of the tumour.
b. The halo is accentuated by compression from the side of the mass on dynamic testing: the echogenic halo does not disappear but remains attached to the nidus. (The compressing fingers have lifted the transducer from the skin so that part of the image is lost.)

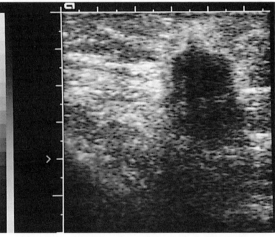
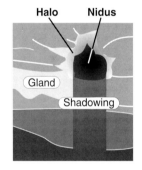

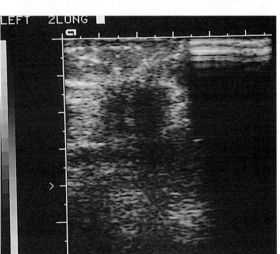
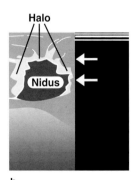

Posterior shadowing is a classical appearance in breast carcinoma (Fig. 9.11.a). It is typically seen in the scirrhous type in which the fibrous stromal tissue predominates. The fibrous tissue absorbs the ultrasound energy more markedly than the surrounding normal tissue and thus gives rise to acoustic shadowing. Characteristically the shadowing is heterogeneous: the irregular distribution of fibrous tissue within the lesion means that some parts attenuate more than others, so that the intensity of the shadowing varies across the lesion, resulting in a vertically banded pattern deep to the mass. Occasionally, in small tumours, the nidus itself is not clear and attenuation may be the only sign drawing attention to the presence of a carcinoma (Fig. 9.11.b). Shadowing of this type must be differentiated from the interface shadows produced by Cooper's ligaments, which are typically seen as fine dark lines that can be traced anteriorly to their origin from the ligaments themselves. Similar shadows from postoperative scar tissue can sometimes be more confusing as they may be wider and originate within the breast parenchyma. In addition, the position of the parenchymal scar need not correspond with the skin incision site. Another cause of intense shadowing is coarse calcification (e.g. from a calcified fibroadenoma or cyst). Here a very bright echo, due to strong reflection, is observed at the surface of the lesion.

Fig. 9.11
Shadowing
a. The majority of carcinomas produce acoustic shadowing (70–80% overall and almost 100% of scirrhous lesions). The irregular shape and halo of this lesion are also typical appearances.
b. With small carcinomas, shadowing may be the only sign of the presence of a tumour. Such narrow shadowing bands must be differentiated from the interface shadows that are commonly produced by Cooper's ligaments or by scar tissue (due to previous surgery). These typically originate from the surface of the glandular tissue whereas shadows from breast carcinomas usually originate from within the glandular tissue itself.

SCF: subcutaneous fat
SL: superficial layer of the superficial fascia

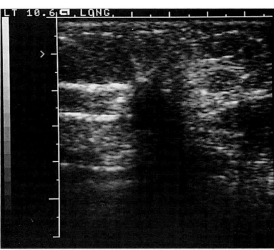

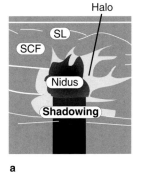

a

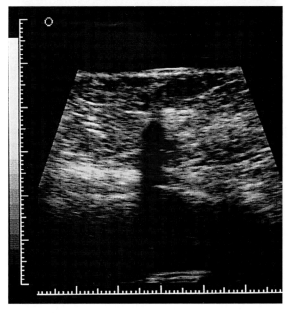

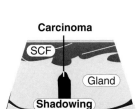

b

Secondary features

Due to their invasive nature, carcinomas often break through normal structures such as the anterior layer of the superficial fascia or the surface of the gland itself, whereas benign lesions do not extend beyond the glandular surface, although they may stretch the overlying tissues smoothly. The ultrasound signs of invasion are particularly useful when a carcinoma is superficially located and they may be apparent even with small tumours when the glandular tissue is atrophic (Fig. 9.12).

Invasive carcinomas may obstruct mammary ducts and cause dilatation of the distal portions. They may also spread within the duct lumina, filling them with echo-poor tumour tissue — the invaded walls are usually irregular. The lumen may also be filled with debris or necrotic material; in this case a bloody nipple discharge is a common feature (Fig. 9.13).

Fig. 9.12
Interruption of surrounding tissues
This small tumour (6 mm) has broken through the surface of the glandular tissue and invaded the subcutaneous fat (arrow). The high D:W ratio and posterior shadowing are also malignant features.

SCF: subcutaneous fat.

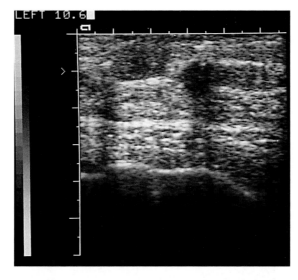
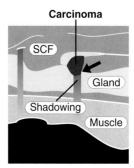

Fig. 9.13
Dilated duct due to malignant spread
Dilatation of a duct central to a lesion ('downstream') cannot be due to obstruction; it indicates ductal invasion which is highly suspicious of malignancy and is often associated with a bloody discharge from the nipple.

GI: mammary gland
RMS: retromammary space
SCF: subcutaneous fat.

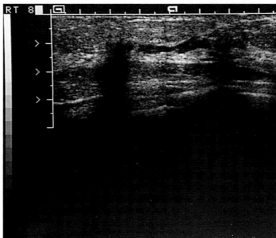
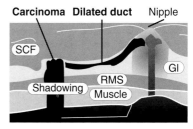

Invasion along Cooper's ligaments causes thickening which may be obvious on ultrasound since normally they are seen only as fine lines (Fig. 9.14). Fibrosis of the ligaments leads to shortening and is the cause of skin dimpling. It produces a stellate pattern on ultrasound.

Invasion into the skin is evidenced by interruption or obliteration of the echogenic line representing the interface between the dermis and subcutaneous fat (Fig. 9.15). The skin itself is often thickened, probably due to oedema consequent upon lymphatic obstruction. In advanced cases, the dilated lymphatics themselves may be visualised (see Ch. 9.5). Invasion to the underlying muscle is well observed on dynamic testing: displacement of the tumour mass pulls the muscle along with it.

Lymphadenopathy due to metastases usually occurs only in advanced cases but is important for staging; the features are described in Chapter 10.1.

Dynamic tests

Typically breast carcinomas are incompressible because of the fibrous tissue they contain. The nidus of a carcinoma does not disappear on compression of the tissue by the probe and the shadowing also persists. Invasion into the surrounding breast tissues makes the mass relatively immobile. These features form the basis of the useful dynamic tests.

Complex cysts and focal forms of benign breast change, two pathologies that may be confused with malignancy, are usually at least moderately compressible. Cysts that have undergone haemorrhage or infection and those containing inspissated material may have an irregular shape and lie proud (high D:W ratio). The focal type of benign breast change may be particularly confusing as the margins of the 'lesion' are irregular and ill-defined. It may also produce distal shadowing; a helpful feature of distinction is that the shadowing from benign breast change reduces or disappears on compression with the probe whereas shadowing behind a carcinoma is persistent.

Mobility is particularly useful in the differentiation of carcinomas from hyalinised fibroadenomas which often cause shadowing and may have a heterogeneous internal texture but do not adhere to the surrounding tissues.

Fig. 9.14
Thickened Cooper's ligaments
Invasion of Cooper's ligaments is seen as echogenic lines at the surface of the tumour. It causes shortening and, consequently, skin dimpling. The radiating pattern gives the ultrasound 'stellate sign'.

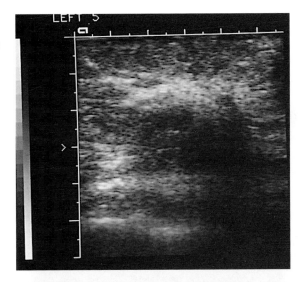

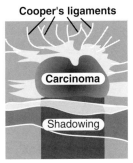

Fig. 9.15
Skin invasion (magnified image)
This carcinoma has directly invaded the skin (arrow), indicated by interruption of the deep echogenic line of the skin, the dermis/subcutaneous fat interface (arrowheads). (Same case as Fig. 8.13)

Gl: mammary gland

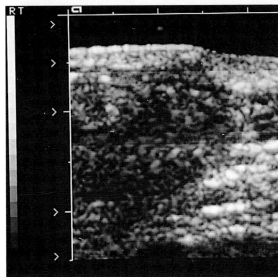

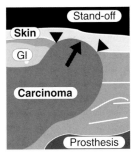

Doppler examination

Doppler signals due to increased vascularity are usually demonstrable within and at the margins of malignant tumours (Plate C.7). Vascularity in a well-circumscribed mass is a suspicious feature, particularly when found in a postmenopausal woman. A knot of abnormal vessels may be a clue to the presence of a mass that is difficult to detect on grey-scale imaging.

Carcinomas without a mass

Carcinomas sometimes do not form a localised mass but spread intraductally or by invasion along the stromal tissues. A small focus of such a tumour is difficult to detect in the heterogeneous breast tissues on ultrasound. This is the predominant reason for false negative ultrasound examinations. Extensive infiltrating (diffuse) lesions may also be difficult to detect, only being evidenced by the architectural distortion they produce and the heterogeneous shadowing and thickening of the glandular or ligamentous tissues that usually accompanies them (Fig. 9.16). Comparison with the surrounding unaffected breast or with the opposite side is helpful but these abnormalities are often difficult to differentiate from benign breast change. Since benign breast change is not usually associated with abnormal vascularity, the demonstration of vascularisation on Doppler raises the suspicion of tumour. Sensitivity is improved by comparing the vascularity with the mirror site in the opposite breast.

Fig. 9.16
Architectural distortion without a mass
The glandular tissue of the right breast is diffusely thickened and produces shadowing, though no actual mass is observed (**a**). These changes are more obvious when compared with the opposite breast (**b**) which has a mottled but normal glandular texture.

SCF: subcutaneous fat
SL: superficial layer of the superficial fascia

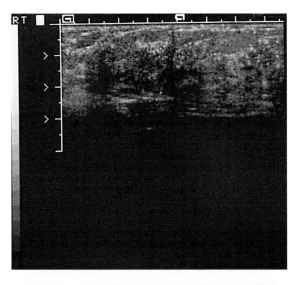
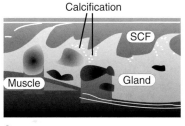
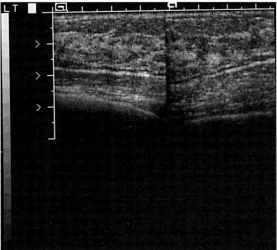
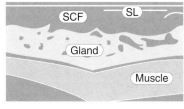

REFERENCES

1. R.W. McDivitt, F.W. Stewart, J.W. Berg: Tumors of the Breast. AFIP, Washington, 1968.
2. E. Silverberg, C.C. Boring, T.S. Squires: Cancer statistics. CA 40; 9–26, 1990.
3. Medical Research Council Annual Report 1988/1989. Medical Research Council Headquarters Office, London, pp 31–32.
4. P. Forrest: Invasive breast cancer. In: Breast Cancer: The Decision to Screen. The Nuffield Provincial Hospitals Trust, London, 1990, pp 26–45.
5. P. Buell: Changing incidence of breast cancer in Japanese–American women. J Nat Cancer Inst 51; 1479–1483, 1973.
6. D. Trichopoulos, B. MacMahon, P. Cole: Menopause and breast cancer risk. J Natl Cancer Inst 48; 605–613, 1972.
7. E.J. Trapido: Age at first birth, parity and breast cancer risk. Cancer 51; 946–948, 1983.
8. UK National Case Control Study Group: Oral contraceptive use and breast cancer risk in young women. Lancet i; 973–982, 1989.
9. K. Hunt, M. Vessey, K. MacPherson, et al: Long-term surveillance of mortality of cancer incidence in women receiving hormone replacement therapy. Br J Obstet Gynaecol 94; 620–635, 1987.
10. G.K. Tokuhata: Morbidity and mortality among offspring of breast cancer mothers. Am J Epidemiol 89; 139–153, 1969.
11. D.E. Anderson, M.D. Badzioch: Risk of familial breast cancer. Cancer 56; 383–387, 1985.
12. D.E. Anderson: Breast cancer in families. Cancer 40; 1855–1860, 1977.
13. C. Cole-Beuglet, R.Z. Soriano, A.B. Kurtz, B.B. Goldberg: Ultrasound analysis of 104 primary breast carcinomas classified according to histologic type. Radiology 147; 191–196, 1983.

9.2 INVASIVE LOBULAR CARCINOMA

CLINICAL FEATURES

The lobular type of invasive carcinoma is the second most common breast malignancy, comprising some 10% of cancers[14,15].

The presentation is the same as for invasive ductal carcinoma, the diagnosis of invasive lobular carcinoma usually being histological. Invasive lobular carcinoma has the same likelihood of axillary node involvement, distant metastasis and survival rate as invasive ductal carcinoma.

A high incidence of bilaterality and multicentricity has been reported with this type of carcinoma, about one quarter of patients having bilateral disease[15,16]. The prognosis is worse in patients with bilateral disease, especially when the two lesions are synchronous[15].

As this type of carcinoma is characterised by a diffuse infiltrating pattern histologically, they may be difficult to detect on mammography, the most common feature being asymmetric density without a definable mass; a dense mass with spiculation is the next most common[17]. Diffuse infiltration may also be seen in metastatic sites such as in the peritoneum and meninges[18].

PATHOLOGICAL FEATURES

Histologically, the tumour is characterised by cells which are identical to those seen in lobular carcinoma in situ: they are small, round and uniform, have a high nucleus/cytoplasm ratio and often contain intracytoplasmic mucin vacuoles. On gross examination the tumour is usually firm, diffuse and poorly defined. The neoplastic cells are usually widely dispersed as single cells or in columns one cell wide known as 'Indian files' (Plate P.9.2). There is thus a considerable amount of intervening stroma which can give rise to diagnostic problems, particularly in small biopsies or frozen sections where the neoplastic nature of the widely dispersed infiltrating cells may not be appreciated. The uncohesive growth pattern is associated with less tissue destruction than is seen in infiltrating ductal carcinomas, the neoplastic cells tending to surround rather than replace normal structures.

The growth pattern of this classical form of infiltrative lobular carcinoma is not present in all cases and three uncommon variants have been described:

1. The alveolar variant[19] in which there are aggregates of 20 or more cells surrounded by collagen
2. The solid variant[20], consisting of sheets of cells with little stroma
3. The tubulolobular type[21] with microtubule formation similar to that seen in tubular carcinoma.

This last variant is said to be associated with a better prognosis.

ULTRASOUND FEATURES

Generally the ultrasound features are similar to those of invasive ductal carcinomas, particularly of the scirrhous type (Fig. 9.17). Invasive lobular carcinomas tend to be highly infiltrative and sometimes do not have a distinct nidus; in some cases only architectural distortion may be demonstrated (Fig. 9.18, see also Fig. 4.22.b, Plate C.7.d). This accounts for some of the false negative results on ultrasound.

Fig. 9.17
Invasive lobular carcinoma
a. The typical ultrasound appearances of breast carcinoma are shown by this invasive lobular carcinoma: an irregular and very echo-poor mass with intense shadowing.
b. This invasive lobular carcinoma is seen as a very ill-defined echo-poor area on ultrasound. Heterogeneous shadowing and a halo around the echo-poor area suggests an infiltrating malignancy.

Ca: carcinoma
Gl: mammary gland
SCF: subcutaneous fat

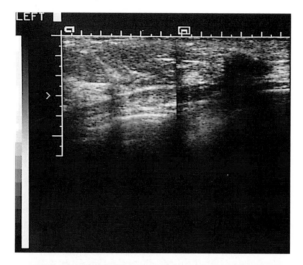
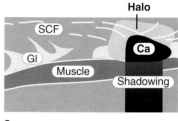

a

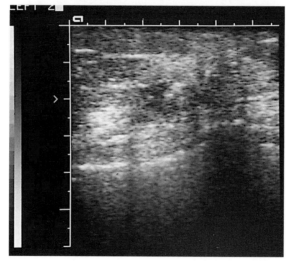
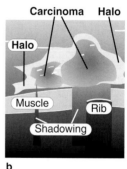

b

REFERENCES

14. J.G. Azzopardi: In situ and invasive lobular carcinoma of the breast. New Frontiers in Mammary Pathology, edited by K.H. Hollmann and J.M. Verley. Plenum Press, New York, 1983, pp 127–145.
15. J.M. Dixon, T.J. Anderson, D.L. Page et al: Infiltrating lobular carcinoma of the breast: an evaluation of the incidence and consequences of bilateral disease. Br J Surg 70; 513–516, 1983.
16. M.L. Lesser, P.P. Rosen, D.W. Kinne: Multicentricity and bilaterality in invasive breast carcinoma. Surgery 91; 234–240, 1982.
17. E.B. Mendelson, K.M. Harris, N. Doshi, H. Tobon: Infiltrating lobular carcinoma: mammographic patterns with pathologic correlation. AJR 153; 265–271, 1989.
18. A. Howell, M. Harris: Infiltrating lobular carcinoma of the breast. Br Med J 291; 1371–1372, 1985.
19. V. Martinez, J.G. Azzopardi: Invasive lobular carcinoma of the breast: incidence and variants. Histopathology 3; H467–488, 1979.
20. R.E. Fechner: Histologic variants of infiltrating lobular carcinoma of the breast. Hum Pathol 6; 373–378, 1975.
21. E.R. Fisher, R.M. Gregorio, C. Redmond, B. Fisher: Tubulolobular invasive breast cancer: a variant of lobular invasive cancer. Hum Pathol 8; 679–683, 1977.

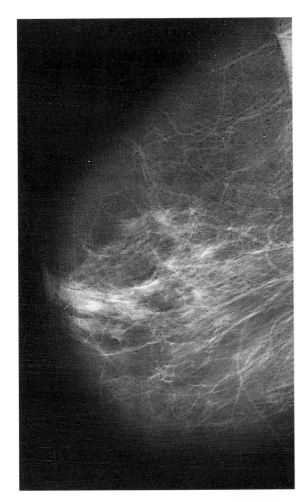
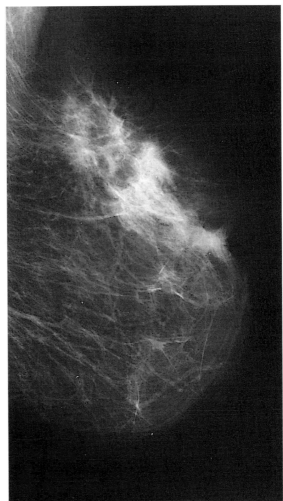

a

Fig. 9.18
Invasive lobular carcinoma
a. On the mammogram, asymmetry with increased density on the left side is obvious by comparison with the opposite side but the tumour mass itself is not clearly seen.
b. On ultrasound, the nidus of this lesion is visualised but is less well-defined than the examples in Figure 9.17. The appearance is best described as 'architectural distortion'. Heterogeneous shadowing is seen.

Gl: mammary gland
IS: interface shadow from Cooper's ligament

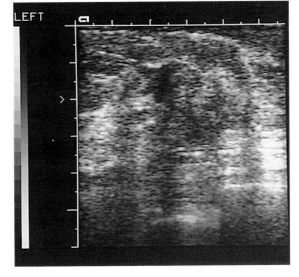

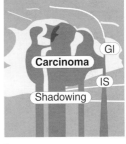

b

9.3 COLLOID CARCINOMA

CLINICAL FEATURES

Colloid carcinoma, variously known as mucinous, mucoid or gelatinous carcinoma, is a rare variety with an incidence of less than 5% of all infiltrating carcinomas. It tends to occur in older women.

Colloid carcinomas can be divided into two types: pure and mixed. Pure colloid carcinomas have slow rate of growth and a relatively good prognosis, while in the mixed type the infiltrative ductal elements determine the prognosis, so they are better classified as 'infiltrating ductal carcinomas with a colloid component'.

Clinically colloid carcinomas tend to be relatively well-delineated and firm but not very hard.

PATHOLOGICAL FEATURES

On naked eye examination, colloid carcinomas are well-circumscribed but not encapsulated and have a pale grey, soft gelatinous cut surface. They are often large. Histologically, they are composed of nests, cords and even isolated cells lying in lakes of extracellular mucin separated by a small amount of fibrous stroma (Plate P.9.3). The tumour cells are relatively small and uniform with only mild or moderate cytological atypia.

ULTRASOUND FEATURES

The ultrasound appearances of colloid carcinomas have a wide variation[22]. In the mixed type the appearances are similar to those of infiltrating ductal carcinomas, depending on the proportion of the elements.

The pure type appear well-circumscribed with relatively well-defined margins and lobulated or knobbly contours (Fig. 9.19). The intensity of the internal echoes is one of the most distinctive features of this type of carcinoma, tending to be almost as echogenic as fatty tissue. This is quite different from the medullary carcinoma, another well-circumscribed carcinoma which is typically very echo-poor. Lesions isoechoic with fatty tissue are uncommon but are particularly difficult to detect because they simulate fat islands or lipomas, especially in involuted breasts in which colloid carcinomas usually occur. This is one of the reasons for failure to visualise a palpable or mammographic mass, especially when using a static scanner. Another difficult differential diagnosis is from fibroadenoma which also may have relatively strong internal echoes and be well-circumscribed. The internal echoes in colloid carcinomas tend to be more heterogeneous and the distal echoes may be enhanced or unchanged.

Evaluation with palpation (dynamic testing) is very useful not only to demonstrate the tumour itself but also to assess its margins and its malignant nature. Colloid carcinomas are harder and less compressible and mobile than fibroadenomas.

Fig. 9.19
Pure colloid carcinoma
a. The echogenicity of this tumour is almost the same as that of the surrounding tissue. It is more reflective than a typical invasive ductal carcinoma. The texture is slightly heterogeneous but the tumour is well-circumscribed and lobulated.

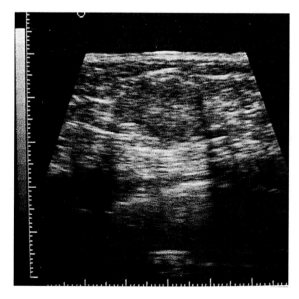

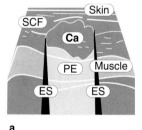

a

REFERENCES

22. H. Sakuma, A. Nagasaki, Y. Fujii, F. Kasumi: Ultrasonographic findings of mucinous carcinoma of the breast. Jap Jnl Med Ultrasonics 12 (suppl I); 169–170, 1985.

b. Mammogram of the same patient. The lobulated outline is more obvious.

c. This patient had a firm palpable mass but on the frozen ultrasound image the mass is difficult to discern because its internal echoes are very similar to those of the adjacent fatty tissue. It was more obvious on dynamic compression testing when its lobulated margin and incompressibility suggested the diagnosis of a colloid carcinoma.

Ca: carcinoma
ES: edge shadow
GI: mammary gland
PE: posterior enhancement
SCF: subcutaneous fat

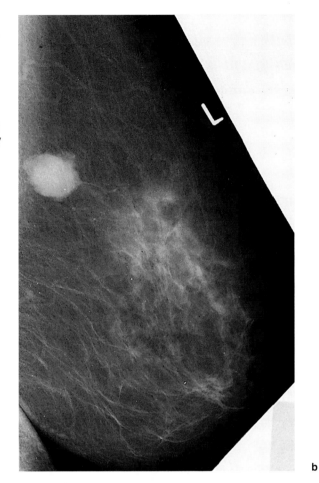

b

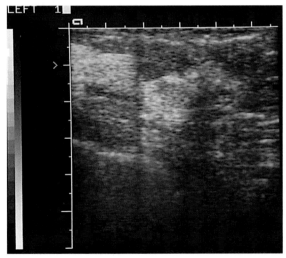

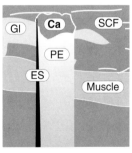

c

9.4 MEDULLARY CARCINOMA

CLINICAL FEATURES

Medullary carcinoma is an uncommon tumour; it has been reported to comprise about 5% of all breast carcinomas but, in some series, the incidence is even lower[23,24]. The average age is about the same as for other carcinomas. The main characteristic of this tumour is its remarkably good prognosis. The 5-year survival is significantly better than for other carcinomas: after 20 years, 74% of patients with operable medullary tumours are alive, compared with 14% of patients with non-medullary carcinomas of similar stage[24]. Host immunity has been suggested as the explanation for this better outlook, and this is consistent with the marked lymphoid infiltration that is often found.

The tumour usually presents as a large but well-circumscribed lump, often located in the periphery of the breast. Skin invasion is rare and ulceration is a late sign. The prognosis remains good even in the presence of axillary node metastases which are not uncommon.

PATHOLOGICAL FEATURES

On macroscopic examination, medullary carcinomas are well-delineated from the surrounding breast (Plate P.9.4), relatively soft in consistency and often large. Histologically, they are composed of cells which, surprisingly in view of the reported better prognosis, show a high grade of cytological atypia and anaplasia with large vesicular nuclei and prominent nucleoli. Necrosis is common and the mitotic rate is often high. No tubular differentiation is seen. The stroma is very scant and consists of fibrous tissue extensively infiltrated by lymphocytes, plasma cells and macrophages.

Some tumours do not conform precisely to the classical histological picture; these may be labelled 'atypical medullary carcinomas' if they show no more than two of the following atypical features:

1. Margins with focal or prominent infiltration
2. Mononuclear infiltrate mild or at tumour margins only
3. Benign appearing nuclei
4. Presence of microglandular features[25].

The survival associated with such tumours has been reported to be better than with ordinary infiltrative ductal carcinomas, though the difference was not statistically significant.

The diagnosis of medullary carcinoma should thus be made only on typical lesions which fulfil the major criteria. As thus defined, the tumour is rare.

ULTRASONIC FEATURES

The ultrasonic appearances of medullary carcinoma typify the pattern seen in circumscribed, cellular carcinomas[26,27]. They are rounded or lobulated in shape with a high D:W ratio. The margins are well defined and generally smooth but they may be slightly irregular due to lobulations and there is no halo. The internal echoes are very weak and slightly heterogeneous; necrosis or haemorrhage may make them more heterogeneous (Fig. 9.20). Calcification is not common. The posterior acoustic enhancement is often marked[28].

On dynamic testing these tumours are mobile but incompressible. Because this is not a common tumour, Doppler studies have not yet been reported.

The same appearances are seen in breast lymphomas and in the variety of invasive ductal carcinomas in which there is little fibrosis. Since medullary carcinomas are rare, homogeneous 'enhancing' tumours detected on ultrasound are more often ductal carcinomas in practice.

REFERENCES

23. R.W. McDivitt, F.W. Stewart, J.W. Berg: Tumors of the breast. AFIP, Washington, 1968.
24. H.J.G. Bloom, W.W. Richardson, J.R. Field: Host resistance and survival in carcinoma of the breast: a study of 104 cases of medullary carcinoma in a series of 1411 cases of breast cancer followed for 20 years. Br Med J 3; 181–188, 1970.
25. R.L. Ridolfi, P.P. Rosen, A. Port, D. Kinne, V. Mike: Medullary carcinoma of the breast: a clinicopathologic study with 10-year follow-up. Cancer 40; 1365–1385, 1977.
26. F. Kasumi, A. Fukami, K. Kuno, T. Kajitani: Characteristic echographic features of circumscribed cancer. Ultrasound Med Biol 8; 369–375, 1982.
27. C. Cole-Beuglet: Sonographic manifestations of malignant breast disease. Semin Ultrasound 3; 51-57, 1982.
28. J.E. Meyer, E. Amin, K.K. Lindfors, et al: Medullary carcinoma of the breast: mammographic and US appearance. Radiology 170; 79–82, 1989.

Fig. 9.20
Medullary carcinoma
a. A slightly lobulated but well-circumscribed mass with heterogeneous internal texture and posterior enhancement are typical features of a medullary carcinoma. However, these features can also be seen in circumscribed ductal carcinomas. (Scan kindly provided by Dr. M. Michell of King's College Hospital, London.)
b. A small medullary carcinoma. The margin is irregular but lacks an infiltrating appearance. Although the lesion is small, its irregular margin and high D:W ratio are malignant features.

ES: edge shadow
GI: mammary gland
PE: posterior enhancement

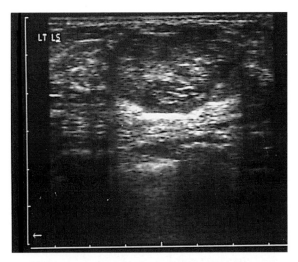

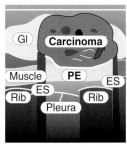

a

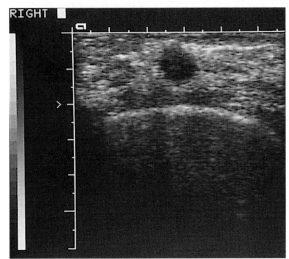

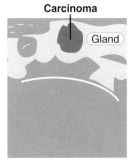

b

9.5 INFLAMMATORY CARCINOMA

CLINICAL FEATURES

Inflammatory carcinoma is a rare but aggressive type of breast carcinoma, comprising 1–3% of all cases[29, 30]. It is often a lethal disease; primary surgery is impractical but the optimum treatment remains controversial — most patients are now treated initially with chemotherapy and radiotherapy[31]. The median survival is only 25–30 months[30, 32].

The diagnosis of inflammatory carcinoma is based on the clinical findings of tenderness, pain and firm enlargement of the breast, together with reddening and oedema of the skin (peau d'orange) affecting more than one-third of the breast[29]. Flattening or retraction of the nipple is a frequent finding and most patients have axillary lymph node metastases by the time of presentation. Bilateral disease is also common, probably due to lymphatic communications across the chest wall. Unlike the common malignancies, a localised mass is palpable in only about one-half of the cases.

Long-standing carcinomas may eventually develop the same appearances, either at the original site or in the opposite breast; strictly these cases should be excluded from the category of inflammatory carcinoma.

PATHOLOGICAL FEATURES

Histologically, most carcinomas associated with this clinical picture are high grade infiltrating ductal carcinomas. The clinical impression of inflammation is not confirmed histologically, there being no inflammatory cell infiltration though some degree of vascular dilatation and oedema may be seen. At least 80% of women with inflammatory carcinoma have demonstrable tumour emboli in dermal lymphatic vessels which are thought to cause the clinical picture (Plate P.9.5)[30]. The explanation for the clinical features in the minority of cases without tumour emboli is not clear: either intralymphatic tumour has been missed through sampling error, or different (and as yet unknown) mechanisms may sometimes apply.

ULTRASOUND FEATURES

Slight skin thickening is the earliest change (Fig. 9.21.a). It is easily missed, partly because the examiner's attention tends to be directed to detecting intraglandular lesions. In addition, evaluation of the subtle skin changes requires the use of a stand-off. When the thickening is focal or uneven, the changes are more readily detectable. Comparison with the opposite breast is useful if slight thickening is suspected. As the skin thickens, the two echogenic lines that are normally demonstrable become less distinct and the skin is seen as a single echogenic layer. With progressive oedema the echogenicity of the skin decreases and it becomes isoechoic with the subcutaneous tissue; in advanced cases, the skin may even become less reflective than the subcutaneous fat (Fig. 9.21.b).

The echogenicity of the subcutaneous fatty tissue may be diffusely increased and its interface with the glandular tissue obscured (Fig. 9.21.b).

Dilated veins are often seen just under the skin layer and lying parallel to it (see Fig. 4.19, Plate C.7.e). Some authors describe visualisation of these veins in the normal breast but, when the ultrasound examination is performed with the patient supine using a hand-held transducer, such veins are only demonstrated when abnormal except occasionally in pregnancy or lactation. Dilated lymphatics are another typical feature of this type of carcinoma; they are seen as branching, anechoic tubular structures in the subcutaneous fatty tissues (Fig. 9.21.c). They can be differentiated from veins by their lack of Doppler signals.

The tumour itself cannot always be demonstrated. If seen, it has the same appearances as an infiltrative ductal carcinoma (Fig. 9.21.d). In cases without a tumour mass, textural distortion of the glandular tissue is usually apparent together with irregular shadowing. This often prevents demonstration of fixation of the glandular tissue to the pectoral muscle which is also common in inflammatory carcinomas.

Axillary lymphadenopathy is a common finding: the examination should include the parasternal, infraclavicular and supraclavicular areas.

Presumably because of the hyperaemia associated with the inflammatory process, these tumours give strong Doppler signals that form spectacular images on colour Doppler in which the lesion and the surrounding breast seem to be alight with an 'inferno' of striking colours (Plate C.7.f). This degree of vascularisation is otherwise only seen with acute infections such as surrounding a breast abscess.

REFERENCES

29. C.D. Haagensen: Diseases of the Breast (3rd edn). W.B. Saunders, Philadelphia, 1986, pp 808–814.
30. C.A. Droulias, C.W. Sewell, M.B. McSweeney, R.W. Powell: Inflammatory carcinoma of the breast: a correlation of clinical, radiologic and pathologic findings. Ann Surg 184; 217–222, 1976.
31. D.L. Ellis, S.L. Teitelbaum: Inflammatory carcinoma of the breast — a pathologic definition. Cancer 33; 1045–1047, 1974.
32. J.N. Fields, C.A. Perez, R.R. Kuske, et al: Inflammatory carcinoma of the breast: treatment results on 107 patients. Int J Radiat Oncol Biol Phys 17; 249–255, 1989.
33. A.U. Buzdar, E.D. Montague, J.L. Barker, et al: Management of inflammatory carcinoma of breast with combined modality approach — an update. Cancer 47; 2537–2542, 1981.

Fig. 9.21
Inflammatory carcinoma

a. The earliest change is skin thickening. In this case the abnormality is best appreciated as non-uniformity of the skin thickness. The glandular tissue is also thickened and produces shadowing; this feature is non-specific if no mass is seen.

b. In this case, there is marked thickening of the skin. The reduced echogenicity of the skin (due to oedema), with the increased echogenicity of the subcutaneous fat, cause inversion of the normal echo contrast between the skin and subcutaneous fat, so that the skin has become less reflective than the subcutaneous fat. Dilated subcutaneous lymphatics are also seen.

c. Markedly dilated lymphatics are seen in this very advanced case. The differentiation between dilated veins and lymphatics is most easily made by colour Doppler; on imaging veins do not usually have branches and they are easily compressible (probably because the cause of dilatation is not obstruction but increased blood flow).

d. A tumour mass is identified in about half of inflammatory carcinomas. No tumour is seen in this case.

Gl: mammary gland
RMS: retromammary space
SCF: subcutaneous fat

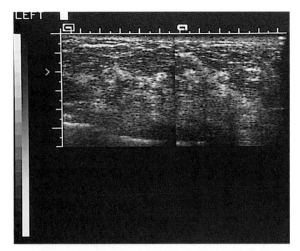
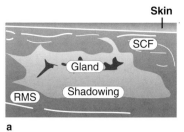
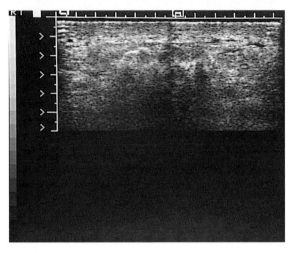
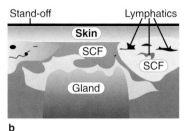
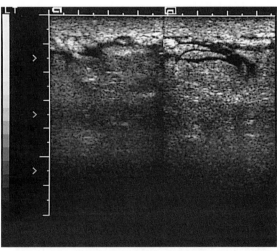
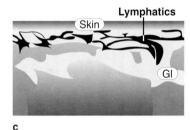
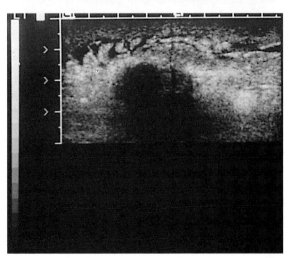
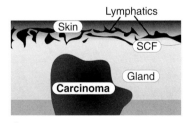

9.6 NON-INVASIVE CARCINOMA (carcinoma in situ)

A carcinoma is defined as non-invasive if there is no stromal invasion. Two types of in situ carcinoma are recognised: ductal (DCIS) and lobular (LCIS).

DUCTAL CARCINOMA IN SITU

CLINICAL FEATURES

Ductal carcinomas in situ (DCIS) may present as a palpable mass of variable size, shape and consistency, depending on the degree of distension and extension along the ductal system and the presence of associated features such as inflammation and fibrosis. Intracystic papillary carcinomas often present as well-demarcated discrete lesions. Nipple discharge is common — spontaneous, persistent, non-lactational, single duct discharge is usually pathological. In such cases where there is no palpable mass, the incidence of carcinoma is reported as around 7%, mostly consisting of DCIS or infiltrative carcinomas with a predominant intraductal component (see Ch. 5.3).

Paget's disease is another presenting pattern with redness or erosion of the nipple, frequently accompanied by itching or a burning sensation. It is generally accepted that Paget's disease is an extension of a breast carcinoma along the ducts into the epidermis and consequently is always associated with an underlying breast carcinoma, though the tumour itself may be subclinical. If the underlying malignancy is purely non-invasive, the prognosis is favourable.

DCIS accounts for a much higher proportion of cases detected at mammographic screening than those presenting with symptoms. Small DCISs are occasionally discovered incidentally in otherwise benign biopsies.

The natural history of DCIS has been difficult to establish as most cases have been treated by mastectomy. It has been estimated that DCIS will progress to invasive carcinoma in about 50% of cases over 10 years if left untreated[34,35]. The recurrence rate after local excision seems to be low, especially if adjuvant radiotherapy is used[36].

PATHOLOGICAL FEATURES

Despite their name, there is now evidence that most ductal carcinomas arise from the terminal duct lobular units[37]. There are several major types which may be intermingled in one lesion.

The solid variety is usually composed of large cells with vesicular nuclei and prominent nucleoli which completely fill the lumina of the lobules and ducts. Central necrosis may occur in this variety, when the term 'comedo carcinoma' may be used. These lesions frequently contain microcalcifications (Plate P.9.6).

Some tumours show a cribriform and/or micropapillary growth pattern; these lesions usually differ cytologically from the solid variant, consisting of smaller cells with hyperchromatic nuclei and a high nucleus/cytoplasm ratio (Plates P.9.7 and P.9.8).

Intracystic papillary carcinomas are papillary carcinomas contained within a cystically dilated duct which has attained a size sufficient to produce a palpable mass.

DCIS may be surrounded by chronic inflammation, fibrosis and elastosis, particularly in the solid and comedo types. There may be extensive spread along the duct sys-

Fig. 9.22
Intraductal carcinoma
No definite mass can be identified on this ultrasound scan over the region where a large (6 cm × 5 cm) mass was palpable The glandular tissue is slightly thickened and heterogeneous and very slight shadowing is seen. The pattern is indistinguishable from benign mammary change and is so subtle that it is easily missed completely. Only increased density was seen on the mammograms. Histologically widespread intraductal carcinoma was found.

Gl: mammary gland
SCF: subcutaneous fat

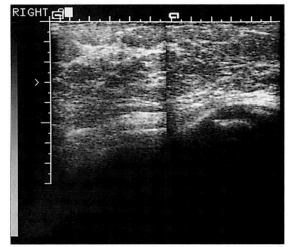

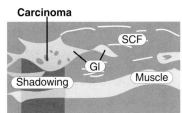

tem to produce a palpable mass. Extension into the lactiferous sinuses and collecting ducts may be followed by infiltration of the epidermis to produce Paget's disease.

Occult foci of invasion may be found in a significant minority of intraduct carcinomas, the incidence depending on the extent of histological sampling. Many cases of metastatic spread from DCIS have been reported; the frequency is difficult to assess but appears to be 1–2%[38–40]. Metastases are presumed to arise from undetected microinvasive foci.

Multicentricity, defined either as foci of tumour more than 5 cm from the main mass, or as tumour in more than one quadrant, occurs in about one-third of patients and is found more frequently with large lesions[40]. It is likely, however, that most cases are due to intramammary spread along the duct system rather than to true multiple sites of origin. Bilateral DCIS is rare.

ULTRASOUND FEATURES

By general consensus the detection and diagnosis of intraductal carcinomas is a difficult problem for ultrasound because they are often small and tend not to form masses.

There are few reports on the ultrasonic appearances of intraductal carcinoma[41] and three patterns have been noted:

1. Masses
2. Architectural distortion
3. Intracystic masses.

The mass in DCIS is an aggregation of involved ducts and so does not form a distinct tumour as is found with an invasive carcinoma. They tend to be more heterogeneous than the masses of invasive carcinomas and the D:W ratios tend to be low.

Architectural distortion is seen in widespread intraductal carcinomas, especially of the comedo type. The glandular tissue of the affected area is usually thickened, echo-poor and heterogeneous, with dilated ducts and calcification. Shadowing may also occur (Fig. 9.22). However, this pattern is also seen in benign mammary change, so that the diagnosis of carcinoma in situ on ultrasound imaging is difficult.

Intracystic tumours, typical of the papillary type, are well-demonstrated on ultrasound as solid elements on the cyst wall. Differentiation from intraductal papilloma is difficult or impossible.

LOBULAR CARCINOMA IN SITU

CLINICAL FEATURES

Because of the difficulty in distinguishing lobular carcinoma in situ (LCIS) from the more severe forms of atypical lobular hyperplasia, some authorities have used the term 'lobular neoplasia'[42].

The lesions are of microscopic size and consequently asymptomatic and non-palpable; they are incidental findings in biopsy specimens. Thus there are no specific diagnostic features of LCIS either clinically, on mammography[43] or on ultrasound.

The clinical importance of LCIS is the high incidence of multicentricity and bilaterality. The incidence depends on the thoroughness of sampling; multicentricity is reported as 70% in mastectomy specimens and bilaterality in biopsy specimens of the contralateral breast as 30%[44]. Up to one-third of patients with LCIS treated by excision biopsy alone subsequently develop invasive carcinoma but, because of the multicentric nature of the disorder, the ipsilateral and contralateral breasts are involved with equal frequency. The invasive tumour tends to appear after a longer time interval than with DCIS, an average of 16 years with a range of 2–31 years after the diagnosis of LCIS having been reported[34]. The hazard rate does not appear to diminish appreciably for at least 25 years.

This complexity makes for difficulties in the management of LCIS. Some favour prophylactic simple mastectomy with axillary dissection (which achieves a complete cure), others simply close observation, while a third option is prophylactic therapy with tamoxifen.

PATHOLOGICAL FEATURES

Pathologically, LCIS differs from DCIS in a number of important respects. The degree of distension of the involved terminal duct lobular unit is slight so that the disease is of microscopic size. The malignant cells are identical to those seen in infiltrating lobular carcinomas, being relatively small and uncohesive and frequently containing intracytoplasmic mucin globules. The growth pattern is always solid and necrosis is absent (Plate P.9.9). Extension into interlobular ducts can occur but the degree of ensuing enlargement is usually slight.

REFERENCES

34. P.P. Rosen, D.W. Braun, D.E. Kinne: The clinical significance of preinvasive breast carcinoma. Cancer 46; 919–925, 1980.

35. D.L. Page, W.D. Dupont, L.W. Rogers, M. Landenberger: Intraductal carcinoma of the breast: follow-up after biopsy only. Cancer 49; 751–758, 1982.

36. S. Schnitt, W. Silen, N.L. Sadowsky, J.L. Connolly, J.R. Harris: Ductal carcinoma in situ (intraductal carcinoma) of the breast. N Engl J Med 318; 898–903, 1988.

37. S.R. Wellings, H.M. Jensen, R.G. Marcum: An atlas of subgross pathology of the human breast with special reference to possible precancerous lesions. J Natl Cancer Inst 55; 231–273,1975.

38. R. Ashikari, S.I. Hajdu, G.F. Robbins: Intraductal carcinoma of the breast (1960–1969). Cancer 28; 1182–1187, 1971.

39. K.C. Westbrook, H.S. Gallager: Intraductal carcinoma of the breast: a comparative study. Am J Surg 130; 667–670, 1975.

40. M.D. Lagios, P.R. Westdahl, F.R. Margolin, M.R. Rose: Duct carcinoma in situ: relationship of extent of noninvasive disease to the frequency of occult invasion, multicentricity, lymph node metastases, and short-term treatment failures. Cancer 50; 1309–1314, 1982.

41. H. Tochio, Y. Konishi, T. Hashimoto et al: Ultrasonographic features of noninvasive breast cancer. Jap Jnl Med Ultrasonics 16 (suppl II); 543–544, 1989.

42. C.D. Haagensen: Diseases of the Breast (3rd edn). W.B. Saunders, Philadelphia, 1986, pp 192–241.

43. T.L. Pope, R.E. Fechner, M.C. Wilhelm et al: Lobular carcinoma in situ of the breast: mammographic features. Radiology 168; 63–66, 1988.

44. R.W. McDivitt, F.W. Stewart, J.W. Berg: Tumors of the Breast. AFIP, Washington, 1968, pp 63–82.

Chapter 10

Malignant disease – local recurrences and metastases

10.1 LYMPH NODE INVOLVEMENT

Lymph node involvement is one of the most important prognostic indicators for breast carcinoma, another being the size of the primary (Fig. 10.1)[1].

The axilla is the commonest site of lymph node involvement. Although tumour size and lymph node involvement have been found to act as independent factors, there is a linear relation between the diameter of the primary tumour and the likelihood of histological lymph node involvement, rising from 30% for tumours < 2 cm, through 50% for tumours 2–5 cm, to 70% for tumours > 5 cm in diameter[1]. Some axillary lymph nodes are palpable: soft, tender lymph nodes are common in women without a breast carcinoma; they are usually due to reactive enlargement and are not suggestive of metastasis. Metastatic lymph nodes are hard and fixed to one another or to other structures. Benign axillary lymph nodes are

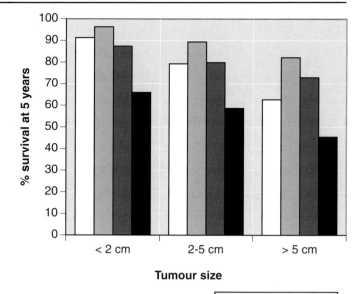

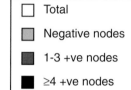

Fig. 10.1
5-year survival rates by size of primary tumour and lymph node status (24 740 cases)

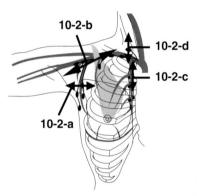

Fig. 10.2
Lymph node metastases
a. Axillary lymph nodes. Multiple round echo-poor nodules with a slightly heterogeneous internal texture are seen in the axillary region. The appearances are typical of metastatic nodes.
b. Level I and II axillary lymph nodes. Lymph nodes low in the axilla (level I) are located superficially and so are often palpable. Because level II lymph nodes lie deep to the pectoralis muscles, they cannot usually be palpated, though they are easily demonstrated on ultrasound.

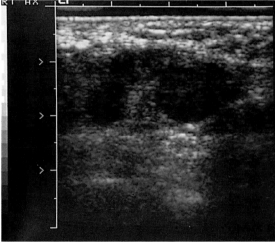

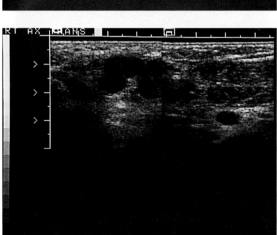

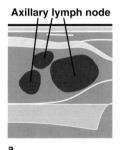

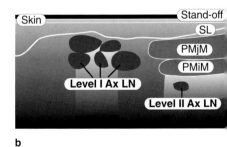

very difficult to demonstrate on ultrasound even if they are palpable, because they are embedded in fatty tissue which has similar echogenicity to the lymph nodes themselves. Occasionally inflammatory enlargement of lymph nodes is seen in women with mastitis as oval echo-poor nodules, each with an echogenic line representing the hilum. Axillary lymph nodes involved with carcinoma are seen as oval, round or lobulated echo-poor masses (Fig. 10.2.a); they are often multiple. Metastatic lymph nodes, as well as inflammatory ones, are often colour Doppler positive (Plate C.13). The internal texture is usually homogeneous but can be heterogeneous in large nodes; microcalcification is not as frequent as in the primary lesions. Ultrasound is particularly useful for level II and III lymph nodes which lie too high in the axilla to be palpated (Fig. 10.2.b). They both have the same appearances as level I metastatic nodes but are seen behind the pectoralis muscles. Ultrasound is reported to be more sensitive in the detection of metastatic axillary lymph nodes than palpation or mammography[2, 3].

The internal mammary lymph nodes are also important as a prognostic indicator (Fig. 10.3)[4,5] and have recently been added to the TNM staging system as N3. As with axillary nodes, involvement of internal mammary nodes correlates with the size of the primary tumour, 16% being involved with tumours < 2 cm while 25% are involved with larger tumours[5]. An association with the patient's age is also reported for internal mammary nodal involvement (the younger the more) but not with the site of the primary. Since internal mammary lymph nodes cannot be palpated, imaging methods are required; lymphoscintigraphy[4], CT (computed tomography)[6,7], or MRI (magnetic resonance imaging) are all effective, but ultrasound is the simplest method. Normal or benign internal mammary lymph nodes are not visualised on ultrasound so that any that are detected almost certainly contain metastatic tumour. They appear as echo-poor nodules in the slightly echo-poor areolar tissue between the costal cartilages in which internal mammary vessels also lie (Fig. 10.2.c), or as focal thickening of that echo-poor space.

c. Metastatic internal mammary lymph node. A small echo-poor nodule is seen in the first intercostal space; normal lymph nodes cannot be detected in this region, so this is almost certainly involved by metastatic disease. This woman had a swollen left breast with redness, the appearances being typical of an inflammatory carcinoma. The primary tumour produced textural distortion with shadowing but no mass could be demonstrated. Multiple axillary lymph node enlargement was also seen.

d. Metastatic supraclavicular lymph node. An oval echo-poor mass is seen in the supraclavicular region. Because lymph nodes are not normally seen in this region, this lesion is probably pathological, most probably metastatic. Differentiation from vessels relies on demonstrating the ovoid shape of nodes compared with the tubular configuration of vessels; the echogenicity is unhelpful because vessels usually contain some echoes, usually reverberation artefact. Demonstrating flow with Doppler confirmed the positions of the vessels.

Ax LN: axillary lymph node
PMiM: pectoralis minor muscle
PMjM: pectoralis major muscle
LN: lymph node
SL: superficial layer of the superficial fascia
V: vessel

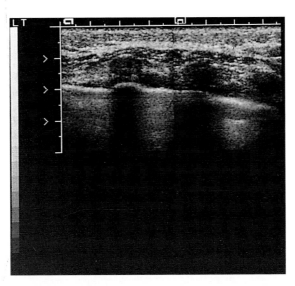

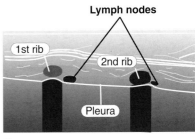

c

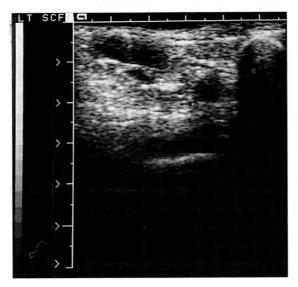

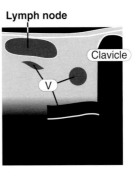

d

They are most commonly found in the upper three or four intercostal spaces, corresponding to the position of perforating branches of the internal mammary vessels supplying the breast. While detection of enlarged lymph nodes in the parasternal region is highly specific for metastasis, the sensitivity is low and visualisation of the area is often difficult in obese women.

Supraclavicular lymph node involvement is usually a late finding. While this area can be palpated, ultrasound is able to find small lymph nodes. No lymph nodes are detected here normally, though cervical lymph nodes are commonly visualised in normal individuals. Almost any malignancy may involve this area and the appearance of lymph nodes is non-specific for the primary site. They are seen as oval, round or lobulated echo-poor masses (Fig. 10.2.d). Differentiation from vessels can be made by following the suspicious areas and confirming they are not tubular or, more directly, with Doppler.

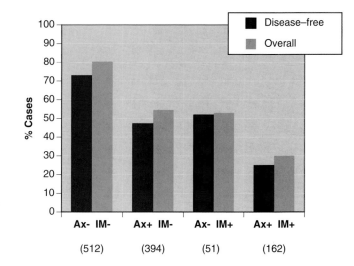

Fig. 10.3
10-year survival of breast cancer patients according to extent of nodal involvement (figures in %)
Survival is markedly reduced when both axillary and internal mammary nodal groups are affected.

Ax–: axillary lymph nodes not involved
Ax+: axillary lymph nodes involved
IM–: internal mammary lymph nodes not involved
IM+: internal mammary lymph nodes involved
( ): number of patients

REFERENCES

1. C.L. Carter, C. Allen, D.E. Henson: Relation of tumor size, lymph node status, and survival in 24,740 breast cancer cases. Cancer 63; 181–187, 1989.
2. J.N. Bruneton, E. Caramella, M. Héry, et al: Axillary lymph node metastasis in breast cancer: preoperative detection with US. Radiology 158; 325–326, 1986.
3. M. Pamilo, M. Soiva, E. Lavast: Real-time ultrasound, axillary mammography, and clinical examination in the detection of axillary lymph node metastases in breast cancer patients. J Ultrasound Med 8; 115–120, 1989.
4. G.N. Ege, R.M. Clark: Internal mammary lymphoscintigraphy in the conservative management of breast carcinoma: an update and recommendations for a new TNM staging. Clin Radiol 36; 469–472, 1985.
5. U. Veronesi, N. Cascinelli, M. Greco, et al: Prognosis of breast cancer patients after mastectomy and dissection of internal mammary nodes. Ann Surg 202; 702–707, 1985.
6. J.E. Meyer, J.E. Munzenrider: Computed tomographic demonstration of internal mammary lymph node metastasis in patients with locally recurrent breast carcinoma. Radiology 139; 661–663, 1981.
7. J.C. Scatarige, E.K. Fishman, E.S. Zinreich, et al: Internal mammary lymphadenopathy in breast carcinoma: CT appraisal of anatomic distribution. Radiology 167; 89–91, 1988.

10.2 METASTASES TO THE BREAST

CLINICAL FEATURES

The breast is an uncommon site of involvement by metastases. Three groups can be recognised[8]:

1. Metastasis from a carcinoma in the opposite breast
2. Metastasis from extramammary primary malignancies (presumed to be blood-borne)
3. Breast involvement in haematological malignancies.

Spread within the same breast may be due to intraductal permeation, or via lymphatics to intramammary lymph nodes in other parts of the breast. Metastasis to the opposite breast usually occurs via lymphatics across the anterior chest wall. Skin thickening is the earliest sign in these cross-lymphatic metastases and is obvious on the mammogram; usually the primary lesion is already far advanced. Skin biopsy is required for confirmation, if necessary. Multicentric origin is believed to be commoner than intramammary spread, though these are difficult to distinguish unless microscopically different histological types or intraductal components that suggest separate primary lesions are found.

Metastases from distant sites are not common. Melanoma, bronchogenic carcinoma (Plate P.10.1), sarcoma and ovarian carcinoma are recognised primary lesions for blood-borne metastasis[8]. Solitary discrete nodules are reported to be the commonest form of presentation; multiple lesions and diffuse involvement are said to be rarer[9], but their incidence is probably underestimated because the multiple or diffuse involvement typical of metastatic disease does not arouse suspicion when seen in advanced primary tumour.

Of the haematological malignancies, lymphoma is the commonest cause of breast involvement (Plate P.10.2). Lymphoma occasionally originates in the breast but in some cases distinguishing primary from secondary involvement is difficult.

ULTRASOUND FEATURES

Because metastasis to the breast is rare, the general appearances are difficult to describe.

Daughter nodules due to intraductal spread of a breast carcinoma usually form close to the primary lesion. Demonstration of dilated ducts suggests ductal spread as the method of extension. Intramammary lymph nodes are most often seen in the upper-outer quadrant of the breast on X-ray mammography but do also occur in all parts of the breast, those in the same quadrant being involved most commonly[10]. The appearances are the same as other metastatic lymph nodes: round, oval or lobulated, well-circumscribed echo-poor masses are seen (see Ch. 10.1).

Skin thickening or blurring of the skin layer of the opposite breast strongly suggests cross-lymphatic metastasis. It is more often seen in the medial or inferior parts of the breast and is less marked in the upper outer quadrants. Invasion of the dermal lymphatics may lead to skin nodules (Fig. 10.4).

Fig. 10.4
Skin metastasis
A well defined homogeneous nodule is seen in the skin layer which is thickened, representing dermal lymphatic invasion. There was an advanced breast cancer in the same breast.

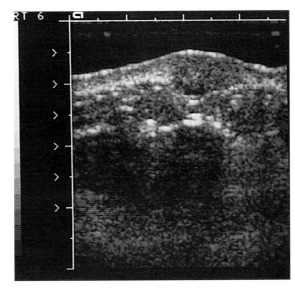
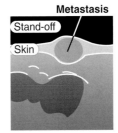

Blood-borne metastases usually form discrete nodules in the breast with minimal local reactive changes or signs of invasion in the surrounding tissues (Fig. 10.5). A metastasis cannot be differentiated from a well-circumscribed breast carcinoma, although multiplicity is suggestive of metastasis. Metastatic melanoma is often highly vascular with obvious flame-like vessels in the tumour on colour Doppler (Plate C.14).

In lymphoma there are two groups of ultrasound features, corresponding to the two patterns on mammography. In one, discrete nodules form which may be solitary or multiple and, because of their uniform cellularity, the internal echoes are extremely low with strong enhancement of the distal echoes. Such lesions are easily misdiagnosed as cysts. The other type is diffuse with widespread thickening of the glandular tissue and a generalised decrease of echogenicity with preservation of the structure of the glandular tissue. The overall appearances are somewhat similar to benign mammary change but more marked (Fig. 10.6). Either one or both breasts can be affected. In both types multiple enlarged lymph nodes are common.

Fig. 10.5
Metastatic melanoma
This large lobulated nodule has very low internal echoes and shows strong posterior enhancement. The high D:W ratio is that of malignancy. The differential diagnosis is between a well-circumscribed carcinoma or a metastatic tumour.

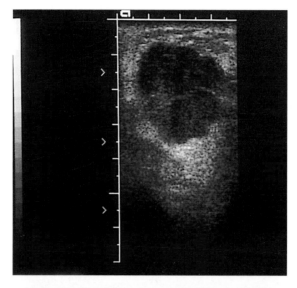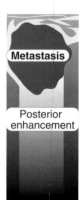

Fig. 10.6
Non-Hodgkin's lymphoma of the breast (diffuse type)
The glandular tissue is diffusely echo-poor. There is no shadowing but the posterior echoes are enhanced. The lesion does not have invasive features and its margin is very ill-defined. This woman had a previous history of lymphoma.

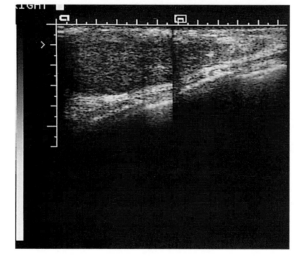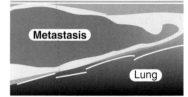

REFERENCES

8. D.D. Paulus, H.I. Libshitz: Metastasis to the breast. Radiol Clin North Am 20; 561–568, 1982.
9. B.D. Toombs, L. Kalisher: Metastatic disease to the breast: clinical, pathologic, radiologic features. AJR 129; 673–676, 1977.
10. R.L. Egan, M.B. McSweeney: Intramammary lymph nodes. Cancer 51; 1838–1842, 1983.

10.3 LOCAL RECURRENCE

CLINICAL FEATURES

Local recurrences after mastectomy usually occur in the skin and so are easily diagnosed clinically, but the wider use of conservative surgery that leaves a significant amount of breast tissue behind has made local recurrence a more difficult diagnostic problem. Local recurrence is relatively uncommon, the incidence in the patients with stage I and II breast carcinoma treated by local excision and radiotherapy being reported as 7% at 5, 14% at 10, and 20% at 20 years[11]. Early detection of local recurrence is important because it is potentially curable.

The findings on palpation are usually the same as in a primary tumour and they may sometimes be easier to detect because of the paucity of breast tissue in the affected region. Occasionally, however, scar tissue or radiotherapy changes (skin thickening or fibrosis of the breast tissue) make physical examination more difficult. Imaging may be valuable in such cases.

Mammography is useful for the detection of local recurrences, especially when they are accompanied by microcalcifications[12], although increased density and scar formation may impair diagnostic accuracy. A valuable feature of mammography is the ease with which it can be compared with a previous study: posttreatment effects do not progress beyond about 6 months, so late enlargement is very suspicious.

ULTRASOUND FEATURES

There are few reports on the diagnostic accuracy of ultrasound for recurrent breast carcinoma. Ultrasound has been reported to be useful[13] but, in fact, scar tissue or fat necrosis sometimes produce appearances indistinguishable from those of breast carcinomas (see Ch. 8).

The ultrasound features of recurrent breast carcinomas depend on whether a mass forms or whether the involvement is diffuse. Recurrent masses have the same appearances as those of primary carcinomas and are seen as localised expansion of the echo-poor line that represents the scar (Fig. 10.7). The shadowing they cause persists under probe compression, unlike scar shadowing which diminishes or even disappears. Diffuse involvement distorts the texture of the breast and usually also causes thickening of the skin, features that are the same as those of an inflammatory carcinoma, though, strictly, this term should only be applied to primary tumours and not to a recurrence (Fig. 10.8). The ultrasound appearances are usually not as striking as the clinical findings of swelling and reddening of the skin.

The literature contains no report on the Doppler features of recurrent breast carcinomas but a vascular mass should be considered as highly suspicious though some recurrent tumours are poorly vascularised, presumably due to radiotherapy effects. Diffuse involvement, like a primary inflammatory carcinoma, is markedly vascular.

Fig. 10.7
Recurrent breast carcinoma
This impalpable mass at the site of previous surgery for breast carcinoma has a definite echo-poor nidus causing shadowing. The high D:W ratio is also a suspicious feature. It proved to be a carcinoma on histology and mastectomy was performed.

DL: deep layer of the superficial fascia
SCF: subcutaneous fat
SL: superficial layer of the superficial fascia

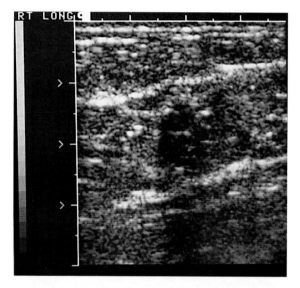
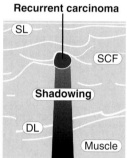

Fig. 10.8
Diffuse recurrence
This woman presented with swelling and redness of the breast after conservation therapy; clinically a recurrence was obvious. The texture of the glandular tissue is diffusely distorted with intense shadowing. Cooper's ligaments are thickened but no discrete mass was seen. The colour Doppler study was strongly positive.

CL: Cooper's ligament
SCF: subcutaneous fat
SL: superficial layer of the superficial fascia

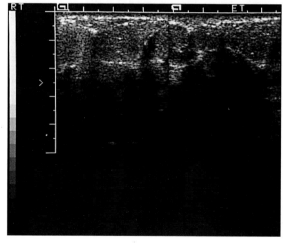
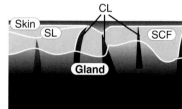

REFERENCES

11. J.M. Kurtz, R. Amalric, H. Brandone, et al: Local recurrence after breast-conserving surgery and radiotherapy; frequency, time course, and prognosis. Cancer 63; 1912–1917, 1989.
12. P.C. Stomper, A. Recht, A.L. Berenberg, et al: Mammographic detection of recurrent cancer in the irradiated breast. AJR 148; 39–43, 1987.
13. W.J. Leucht, D.R. Rabe: Sonographic findings following conservative surgery and irradiation for breast carcinoma. Ultrasound Med Biol 14 (suppl 1); 27–41, 1988.

10.4 METASTASES FROM BREAST CARCINOMA

The presence of any distant metastasis (including ipsilateral supraclavicular lymph node involvement) classifies the patient as Stage IV with a correspondingly worse prognosis. The skeleton is the commonest site for distant metastasis and is conventionally investigated by radioisotope bone scanning, though NMR (nuclear magnetic resonance) scans may prove to be more sensitive (Fig. 10.9)[14,15]. Ultrasound is routinely used to evaluate and follow metastases in the abdomen. Typical cases and problems are described in this chapter.

The commonest use of ultrasound in staging and follow-up of patients with breast carcinoma is for liver metastases, but evaluation of the adrenal glands and upper para-aortic lymph nodes as well as for pleural and pericardial effusions and ascites should all be performed. The ovaries can be scanned at the same time if the patient has a full bladder or, as a separate study, via the transvaginal route. Sector or curved linear arrays operating at 3–5 MHz are suitable for abdominal scanning. Although ultrasound has a relatively high sensitivity for detecting abnormalities, the appearances are often nonspecific; for example, metastases from other malignancies cannot be distinguished and coexistent benign abnormalities have confusingly similar appearances. Biopsy under ultrasonic guidance may be required for histological confirmation.

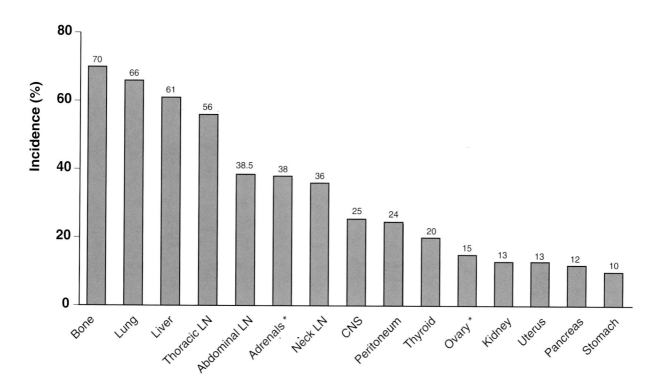

Fig. 10.9
Sites of metastases (647 autopsies in primary breast carcinoma)
* Excluding adrenalectomised or ovariectomised patients.

LIVER METASTASES

There are several reports on the detectability of liver metastases, mostly comparing CT with ultrasound[16]. Ultrasound is usually chosen first because of its availability, cost-effectiveness and non-invasiveness. Its sensitivity greatly depends on the patient's build: in obese patients, high attenuation and dispersion of the ultrasound beam by subcutaneous fat tend to degrade the images. A liver located high under the rib cage makes the examination technically difficult such that portions may be inaccessible. Another factor which decreases the sensitivity of ultrasound is fatty change of the liver; though commonly associated with obesity, it can also be caused by hepatotoxic drugs such as antimitotics. The ultrasonographic appearances of fatty liver include high reflectivity (the 'bright liver') and strong attenuation of the sound beam. The former sometimes helps in the detection of superficially located small echo-poor lesions by increasing their contrast with the liver, but the increased attenuation causes poor visualisation of the deep areas; CT is superior in these patients.

Echo-poor nodules are the commonest manifestation of metastatic deposits from breast carcinoma (Fig. 10.10.a). If they are multiple there is no difficulty in the diagnosis, but a single lesion is less diagnostic. When small echo-poor lesions occur in a fatty liver, they are easily misinterpreted as cysts. This is partly because of their low echoes by contrast with the increased echogenicity of the liver parenchyma (so that gain is set lower than usual), but also because these lesions may show posterior enhancement (the TGC is set for the strongly attenuating liver and is inappropriately high for the deposit, so that they show enhancement).

The 'target' or 'bull's eye' pattern, in which an iso-echoic or slightly echogenic nodule is surrounded by an echo-poor band, may be seen occasionally (Fig. 10.10.b). (Note that this echo-poor 'halo' is the reverse of the strongly reflective halo typically seen around primary breast cancers.) This pattern is more frequent in metastases from the gastrointestinal tract or lung.

Liver metastases from breast carcinoma may occasionally be strongly reflective (Fig. 10.10.c). When they are multiple or intermingled with echo-poor nodules or when they develop during follow-up scans, the diagnosis of metastases is straightforward. The relatively rare solitary echogenic deposits are difficult to differentiate from haemangiomas; helpful features suggestive of haemangioma are the more intense echoes without shadowing and the absence of mass effects. Haemangiomas do not have a halo. Echogenic metastases are more common in secondaries from mucin-producing adenocarcinomas, typically carcinomas of the gastrointestinal tract or ovary, and they often calcify.

Cystic deposits are particularly problematical for ultrasound as they simulate benign cysts; most commonly encountered with ovarian and gastric primaries, they are also occasionally found in breast carcinoma. Biopsy or serial studies are needed to establish the diagnosis.

Diffuse involvement is another pattern which is sometimes seen, especially in metastases from breast carcinomas (Fig. 10.10.d). If the whole liver is affected, the diagnosis can be difficult because there is no remaining normal tissue to provide background against which the lesion can be detected. Decreased echogenicity, coarsening of the texture and hepatomegaly are usually seen. Vessels, especially hepatic veins, may be compressed by the extensive tumour. The decreased reflectivity can be evaluated by comparison with the kidneys or spleen, which normally have almost the same or slightly less intense echoes than liver. Comparison should only be made between areas at the same depth (because of the unpredictable effects of attenuation) and is valid only when the kidneys and spleen are normal. With such extensive metastases, the liver function tests are usually abnormal. CT or liver biopsy may be required to confirm the diagnosis.

Fig. 10.10
Liver metastases
a. Echo-poor metastases. Echo-poor nodules are the commonest pattern of metastatic deposits to the liver. (Coronal scan.)
b. 'Target' or 'bull's eye' metastases. The 'target' or 'bull's eye' pattern produced by an echo-poor band around the lesion may occur in metastatic deposits from carcinoma of the breast. The echo-poor appearance of this 'halo' is different from that around a primary breast carcinoma where it is echogenic. In this patient, echo-poor deposits without a halo are also seen. (Intercostal scan.)
c. Echogenic metastases. Occasionally, metastatic deposits from carcinoma of the breast are strongly reflective, though this pattern is commoner from the gastrointestinal tract or ovary. This lesion is very similar in appearance to a haemangioma but the diagnosis was clear as it developed during follow-up and eventually became echo-poor. (Transverse scan.)
d. Diffuse metastases. Liver metastases from breast carcinoma are sometimes diffuse and do not form discrete masses. Hepatomegaly, a heterogeneous or coarsened texture and mass effects (e.g. vessel compression) are usually seen. (Longitudinal scan.)

GB: gall bladder
IVC: inferior vena cava
PV: portal vein

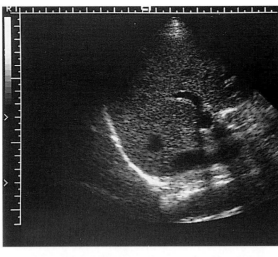
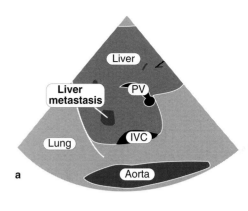
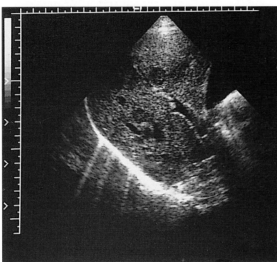
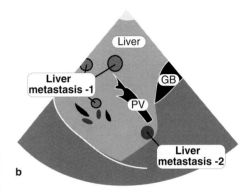
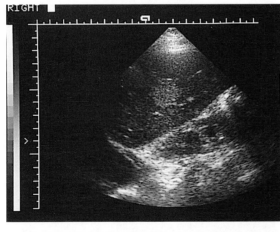
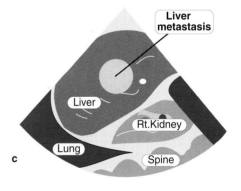
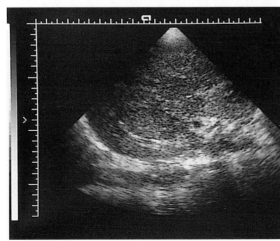
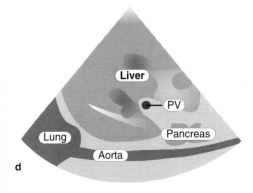

ADRENAL METASTASES

Metastatic deposits from breast cancer to the adrenal glands are common and often bilateral. Because the liver acts as an acoustic window, the right adrenal is easier to visualise on ultrasound than the left which is often obscured by bowel gas (especially the stomach). Affected adrenal glands are enlarged and usually echo-poor (Fig. 10.11.a). As they enlarge further, they tend to become heterogeneous with cystic areas due to necrosis (Fig. 10.11.b). Adrenal function is rarely impaired, even when both glands are involved.

PARA-AORTIC LYMPH NODE METASTASES

Upper para-aortic lymph node involvement in breast cancer is rare by comparison with their frequent involvement in abdominal malignancies, and is usually found only in late stage disease. Echo-poor rounded or lobulated masses are seen (Fig. 10.12).

OVARIAN METASTASES

The incidence of ovarian metastasis is about 15% in autopsy series but they are much more commonly demonstrated on histological studies of oophorectomy specimens when it is reported in some 25% of cases[17]. Macroscopic metastasis detected by ultrasound is not common: they are often bilateral and may obstruct a ureter, causing hydronephrosis. Transvaginal ultrasound using a high frequency transducer (5–7.5 MHz) improves the visualisation of the ovaries and allows earlier detection (Fig. 10.13).

Fig. 10.11
Adrenal metastasis
a. The normal adrenal glands may be visualised as thin (<5 mm) echo-poor linear structures but they are not always identified. Thickened or nodular adrenal glands are abnormal and most commonly are due to metastases. In this case, an echo-poor liver metastasis is also seen. (Transverse scan.)
b. Adrenal metastasis with necrosis. Cystic changes, probably due to necrosis, may occur in advanced cases. The adrenal mass becomes heterogeneous. (Intercostal scan.)

IVC: inferior vena cava

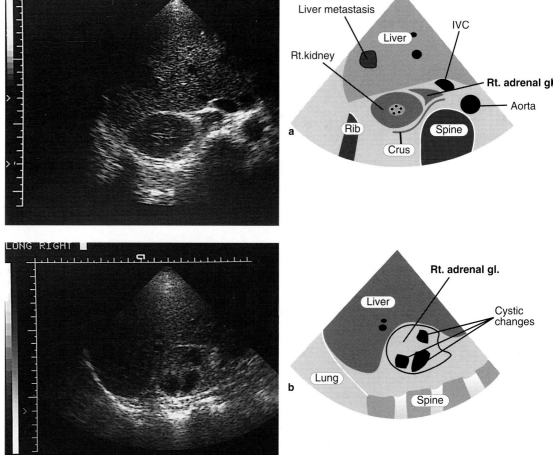

Fig. 10.12
Para-aortic lymph node metastases
Small echo-poor nodules are seen both sides of the inferior vena cava. Abdominal lymph node enlargement is not common in breast carcinoma. (Same patient as Fig.10.11.b.) (Transverse scan.)

IVC: inferior vena cava
LN: lymph node
P: pancreas
PV: portal vein

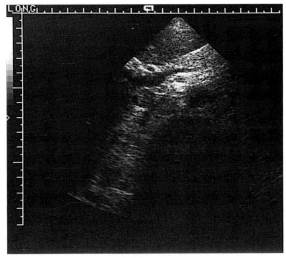
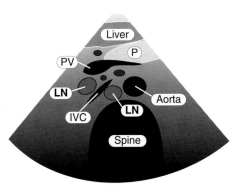

Fig. 10.13
Ovarian metastasis (Kruckenberg tumour)
An enlarged right ovary is seen on this transabdominal scan (**a**, transverse scan); the lobulated shape and heterogeneity are better seen on the transvaginal scan (**b**). This tumour compressed the ureter, causing a right hydronephrosis.

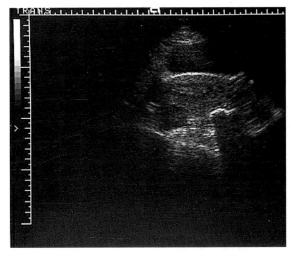
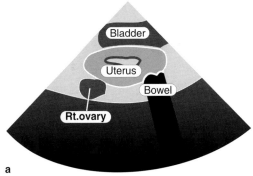

a

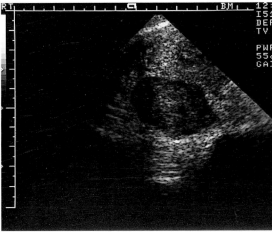
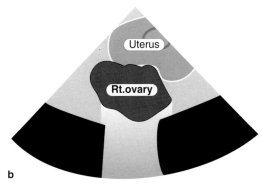

b

ASCITES

Ascites is a late feature, usually seen in patients with multiple widespread metastases. Even a small amount of ascites can be detected by ultrasound as an echo-free crescent in Morrison's pouch at the site of the peritoneal reflection between the liver and the right kidney (Fig. 10.14).

PLEURAL EFFUSIONS

Small pleural effusions can be detected by ultrasound in the posterior costophrenic recess (Fig. 10.15.a). Masses in the pleural space may also be seen (Fig. 10.15.b).

Fig. 10.14
Ascites
Ultrasound is sensitive to very small amounts of ascites. A fine echo free line separating the liver from the right kidney indicates a trace of ascites in Morrison's pouch.

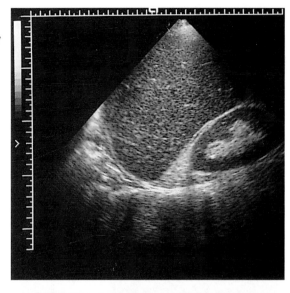
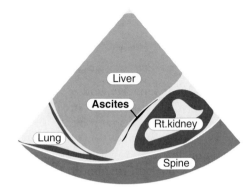

Fig. 10.15
Pleural involvement
a. Pleural effusion. A small amount of pleural fluid is well seen on ultrasound in the posterior costophrenic recess. (Intercostal longitudinal scan.)
b. Pleural effusion with a mass. A metastatic pleural mass is shown, together with a pleural effusion. The effusion is not completely echo-free especially in the posterior part, suggesting debris or blood-stained contents. (Intercostal longitudinal scan.)

D: diaphragm
HV: hepatic vein

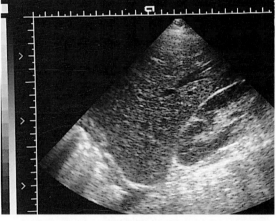
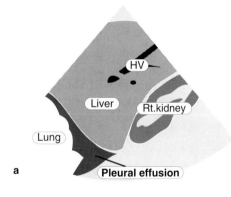

a

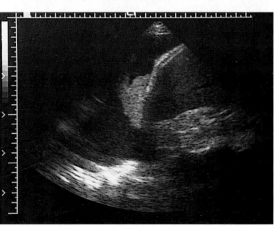
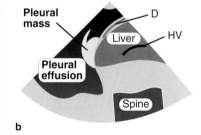

b

REFERENCES

14. E. Viadana, I.D.J. Bross, J.W. Pickren: An autopsy study of some routes of dissemination of cancer of the breast. Br. J. Cancer 27; 336–340, 1973.
15. C. Kamby, I. Vejborg, B. Kristensen, et al: Metastatic pattern in recurrent breast cancer—special reference to intrathoracic recurrence. Cancer 62; 2226–2233, 1988.
16. P.O. Alderson, D.F. Adams, B.J. McNeil et al: Computer tomography, ultrasound, and scintigraphy of the liver in patients with colon or breast carcinoma: a prospective comparison. Radiology 149; 225–230, 1983.
17. C.D. Haagensen: Diseases of the Breast (3rd edn). W.B. Saunders, Philadelphia,1986, p 709.

The current TNM system used for classification and staging of breast carcinoma is that approved by both the American Joint Committee on Cancer (AJCC) and the Union Internationale Contre le Cancer/TNM Committee (UICC/TNMC). Achieving a worldwide agreement on staging has been a protracted process that began in the 1920s leading to the introduction of the TNM concept for the classification of malignancy during the decade 1943–1952. In 1954 the UICC initiated activities on the clinical staging of cancer based on the TNM classification which was defined as: T for the extent of the primary tumour, N for the extent of regional lymph node metastases, and M for absence or presence of distant metastases. In 1982 the national TNM committees began to formulate a universal classification and staging system; after much debate, international agreement was achieved in 1986 with the approval of all national TNM committees[18]. This classification and staging system was published by the UICC in 1987[19] and the AJCC in 1988[20].

The principle of the TNM system is to classify tumours by their anatomic extent using the TNM categories, and then to group combinations of the TNM into prognostically similar categories, called stages. The general principles of staging are as follows:

Stage 0 = carcinoma in situ
Stage I = localised cancer
Stage II = limited local or regional spread
Stage III = extensive local or regional spread
Stage IV = distant spread

The purposes of the TNM classification and staging are:

1. To select appropriate standard treatments
2. To evaluate the results of new treatments
3. To acquire data in an ordinary fashion for statistical analysis of end-results
4. To estimate prognosis.

Furthermore, data throughout the world should be comparable.

TNM CLASSIFICATION

The TNM classification is divided into clinical staging (T, N and M, more correctly termed cT, cN, cM) and pathological staging (pT, pN, pM).

Clinical staging includes physical examination (inspection and palpation) together with pathological tests to establish the diagnosis of breast carcinoma, requiring only a small amount of tissue for histology. Appropriate operative findings are important components of clinical staging; these include the size of the primary tumour and the presence or absence of chest wall invasion and of regional or distant metastases.

Pathological staging includes:

1. All data used for clinical staging.
2. Surgical resection and pathological resection of :
a. The primary carcinoma, including not less than excision of the lesion with no tumour in any margin of resection by gross pathological examination. (A case can be staged pathologically if there is microscopic but no gross involvement at the margin. If there is tumour in the margin of resection on gross inspection, it is coded TX.)
b. Resection of at least the lower axillary lymph nodes, i.e. those located lateral to the lateral border of the pectoralis minor muscle (level I). Such a resection will usually include six or more lymph nodes.

T (primary tumour) classification

TX. Primary tumour cannot be assessed.
T0. No evidence of primary tumour.
Tis. Carcinoma in situ:
Clinical Paget's disease of the nipple with no tumour mass.
Pathological intraductal carcinoma, lobular carcinoma in situ, or Paget's disease with no invasive component.
T1. Tumour 2.0 cm or less in greatest dimension.
T1a. ≤ 0.5 cm
T1b. $> 0.5, \leq 1.0$ cm
T1c. $> 1.0, \leq 2.0$ cm
T2. Tumour more than 2.0 cm but not more than 5.0 cm in greatest dimension.
T3. Tumour more than 5.0 cm in greatest dimension.
T4. Tumour of any size with direct extension to chest wall or skin. Chest wall includes ribs, intercostal muscles, and serratus anterior muscle but not pectoral muscle since fixation to the pectoral fascia does not influence staging.
T4a. Extension to chest wall.
T4b. Oedema (including peau d'orange) or ulceration of the skin of the breast, or satellite skin nodules confined to the same breast.
T4c. Both a and b above.
T4d. Inflammatory carcinoma*.

The measurement used for clinical classification of the primary tumour (cT) is the one judged to be the most accurate (e.g. physical examination or the mammogram).

---

* Inflammatory carcinoma is a clinicopathological entity characterised by diffuse brawny induration of the skin of the breast with an erysipeloid edge, usually without an underlying palpable mass. Radiologically there may be a detectable mass and characteristic thickening of the skin over the breast. This clinical presentation is due to tumour embolisation of dermal lymphatics. (See Ch. 9.5.)

The tumour size used for pathological classification (pT) is the invasive component. For example, if there is a large in situ component (e.g. 4.0 cm) and a small invasive tumour (e.g. 0.5 cm), the tumour is classified as T1a, as though its total extent were 0.5 cm. The size of the tumour should be measured before any tissue is removed for special studies such as oestrogen receptor assays.

When there are multiple simultaneous tumours, only the measurement of the largest mass is used for classification (T), and the record is entered as a case of 'multiple simultaneous ipsilateral primary carcinomas'. Such cases should be analysed separately. Simultaneous bilateral breast carcinomas are also staged separately as 'independent primary carcinomas'.

Paget's disease with a demonstrable mass (clinical) or an invasive component (pathological) is classified according to the size of the tumour mass or invasive component.

Dimpling of the skin, nipple retraction, or any other skin change except those described under inflammatory carcinoma (T4b) may occur in T1, T2, or T3 without changing the classification.

N (regional lymph nodes) clinical classification

NX. Regional lymph nodes cannot be assessed (e.g. previously removed, or not available for pathological study).

N0. No regional lymph node metastasis.

N1. Metastasis to movable ipsilateral axillary lymph node(s).

N2. Metastasis to ipsilateral axillary lymph nodes, fixed to one another or to other structures.

N3. Metastasis to ipsilateral internal mammary lymph node(s).

Involvement of intramammary lymph nodes is considered as equivalent to axillary nodes for staging purposes.

Metastases to any other lymph nodes are considered as distant (M1); this includes supraclavicular, cervical and contralateral internal mammary node groups.

pN (regional lymph nodes) pathological classification

pNX. Regional lymph nodes cannot be assessed (e.g. previously removed or not removed for pathological study).

pN0. No regional lymph node metastasis.

pN1. Metastasis to movable ipsilateral axillary lymph node(s).

pN1a. Only micrometastases (< 0.2 cm).

pN1b. Metastasis to lymph node(s) > 0.2 cm.

pN1bi. Metastasis in one to three lymph nodes > 0.2 cm and all < 2.0 cm in greatest dimension.

pN1bii. Metastasis to four or more lymph nodes, any > 0.2 cm and all < 2.0 cm in greatest dimension.

pN1biii. Extension of tumour beyond the capsule of lymph node metastasis < 2.0 cm in greatest dimension.

pN1biv. Metastasis to a lymph node ≥ 2.0 cm in greatest dimension.

pN2. Metastasis to ipsilateral axillary lymph nodes that are fixed to one another or to other structures.

pN3. Metastasis to ipsilateral internal mammary lymph node(s).

M (distant metastasis)

MX. Presence of distant metastases cannot be assessed.

M0. No distant metastasis.

M1. Distant metastasis present (includes metastasis to ipsilateral supraclavicular lymph node(s)).

Stage grouping

The stage grouping using TNM categories is shown in Table 10.1.

G (histopathologic grading)

GX. Grade of differentiation cannot be assessed.

G1. Well-differentiated.

G2. Moderately differentiated.

G3. Poorly differentiated.

G4. Undifferentiated.

THE TNM CLASSIFICATION AND ULTRASOUND EXAMINATION

The clinical TNM classification is based on clinical examination (inspection and palpation), to which the use of mammography for size measurements has recently been added (third edition). Strictly ultrasound does not add to this.

However, ultrasound measurements can be useful for impalpable and mammography negative carcinomas. Although ultrasound measurements correspond well with the histological sizes[21], the difference of the sizes between

Table 10.1 TNM Staging			
Stage 0	Tis	N0	M0
Stage I	T1	N0	M0
Stage IIA	T0	N0	M0
	T1	N1*	M0
	T2	N0	M0
Stage IIB	T2	N1	M0
	T3	N0	M0
Stage IIIA	T0	N2	M0
	T1	N2	M0
	T2	N2	M0
	T3	N1,N2	M0
Stage IIIB	T4	Any N	M0
	Any T	N3	M0
Stage IV	Any T	Any N	M1

* The prognosis of patients with pN1a is similar to that of patients with pN0.

palpation and ultrasound may cause confusion if they are intermixed and ultrasound has not been accepted as a replacement for clinical measurement of palpable masses. Problems remain in special situations (e.g. measurement of an intracystic mass).

As conservative therapy becomes more widely used, accurate clinical staging has become more important. Metastatic axillary lymph nodes are more reliably identified on ultrasound than by clinical examination[22,23]. Chest wall invasion can be assessed more precisely, in particular using dynamic tests. In addition, ultrasound can add information which cannot be obtained by palpation (e.g. parasternal and level II and III axillary nodes, which are not palpable, can be visualised on ultrasound). The accuracy of these relatively new applications of breast ultrasound has not yet been fully evaluated.

REFERENCES

18. R.V.P. Hutter: At lást — worldwide agreement on the staging of cancer. Arch Surg 122; 1235–1239, 1987.
19. P. Hermanek, L.H. Sobin: UICC TNM Classification of Malignant Tumours (4th edn). Springer-Verlag, Berlin, 1987.
20. Manual for Staging of Cancer (3rd edn), edited by O.H. Beahrs, D.E. Henson, R.V.P. Hutter, M. Myers. J.B. Lippincott, Philadelphia, 1988.
21. B.D. Fornage, O. Toubas, M. Morel: Clinical, mammographic, and sonographic determination of preoperative breast cancer size. Cancer 60; 765–771, 1987.
22. J.N. Bruneton, E. Caramella, M. Hery, et al: Axillary lymph node metastases in breast cancer: preoperative detection with US. Radiology 158; 325–326, 1986.
23. M. Pamilo, M. Soiva, E. Lavast: Real-time ultrasound, axillary mammography and clinical examination in the detection of axillary lymph node metastases in breast cancer patients. J Ultrasound Med 8; 115–120, 1989.

Chapter 11

Indications for breast ultrasound

DIAGNOSTIC ACCURACY OF BREAST ULTRASOUND

The sensitivity and specificity of breast ultrasound have been the subject of several studies, in many of which ultrasound has been compared with other modalities (Table 11.1). The accuracy of each depends on many factors. The skill of the examiners is probably the most important, especially for ultrasound, because there are no objective criteria that completely differentiate between malignant and benign lesions in any modality; the size of the mass (especially whether a screening population is included) and the quality of the equipment are also significant factors. In addition, there may be a bias towards one technique because few people apply all modalities to every patient and interpret them independently; information derived from other examinations (e.g. on the location of a mass) facilitates the diagnosis on ultrasound and mammography while location of an impalpable mammographic abnormality may expedite finding the lesion on ultrasound. The indications for biopsy differ between hospitals and many cases of benign disease have to be excluded from analysis because of lack of histological confirmation. Generally, for palpable carcinomas, an abnormality is detected by ultrasound in more than 95% of cases, with identification of the tumour in about 90%, giving a sensitivity (diagnosis as malignancy) of 80–90%.

INDICATIONS FOR BREAST ULTRASOUND

The four most commonly used diagnostic methods for breast disease are palpation (including inspection), mammography, ultrasound and fine needle aspiration cytology (FNAC). Combining several diagnostic modalities increases sensitivity for malignancy[8], but not only does this decrease specificity (number of false positives) but it also adds to expense. It is important to be aware of the strengths and weak points of each modality to make the most effective choice for each patient.

Some advantages of ultrasound include:

1. The examination is completely non-invasive: not only is it free from ionising radiation (so it can be used without restriction, for example in the young and pregnant and even in children) but, because it does not require compression, it is well-tolerated in inflammatory conditions and immediately after surgery.

2. Ultrasound images are tomograms of the breast in contradistinction to palpation or X-ray mammography, in which the whole thickness of the breast is examined together. Because of this the anatomical information is more precise on ultrasound while the use of real-time enables the exact localisation of a mass or of the needle tip during interventional procedures to within a few millimetres.

3. Ultrasound is extremely reliable in differentiating cystic from solid lesions.

Table 11.1 Sensitivity and specifity of ultrasound (in comparison with other modalities)

	Total no. of cases	Ultrasound Sensitivity %	Ultrasound Specificity %	Mammography Sensitivity %	Mammography Specificity %	Palpation Sensitivity %	Palpation Specificity %	Technique
Sickles et al[1] (1982)	64*	58	–	97	–	–	–	Static
Schmidt et al[2] (1983)	268 (97*)	90	72	93	–	–	–	
Egan et al[3] (1984)	297 (107*)	72	94	88	78	69	36	Static
Kopans et al[4] (1985)	127*	64	–	94	–	91	–	Static
Smallwood et al[5] (1986)	142	91	81	81	69	–	–	Static
Tohno et al[6] (1986)	528 (131*)	75	92	69	92	81	88	Static & real-time
Hayashi et al[7] (1988)	148 (45*)	87	90	–	–	–	–	Real-time, Palpable masses
Van Dam et al[8] (1988)	201	78	89	94	55	88	71	Static & real-time, Palpable masses
Dempsey[9] (1988)	252*	88	–	–	–	–	–	
Leucht et al[10] (1988)	755	94	77	95	49	90	64	Real-time

(* Number of carcinomas).

On the other hand, there are some important limitations which must be kept in mind:

1. Ultrasound images represent the acoustic characteristics of the tissue whereas palpation senses differences of consistency and mammography differences in X-ray absorption; none correlates exactly with the changes demonstrated on histology. Different histological tissues may have the same ultrasound appearances if their acoustic characteristics are identical, and vice versa.

2. The resolution of the images has improved greatly over the past decade but is still not as good as X-ray mammography.

The indications for ultrasound mammography are still developing; it is most commonly used when more information about indeterminate breast abnormalities is required. At present it does not have a primary role in screening though it is valuable in the assessment of abnormalities detected by the screening process. The current indications are summarised in Table 11.2.

Evaluation of palpable abnormalities

Ultrasound is not indicated for women whose breasts are entirely normal on palpation because it rarely detects non-palpable carcinomas (7/62 carcinomas reported by Sickles et al, all of which were also detected on mammography[1], none in the series of 127 carcinomas reported by Kopans et al[4]). This also raises the question of whether the examination should be confined to the lesion or should include the whole breast and the opposite side also. Strictly, the extended examination is not necessary but it is usually performed because, occasionally, breast carcinomas without a mass can be diagnosed by asymmetry of the breast texture on ultrasound. In addition, one abnormality may mask another, so that preferably the whole breast should be checked in the course of the preoperative evaluation to exclude multicentric lesions.

Palpable abnormalities may be considered in several groups as follows:

Lumpy breasts

Ultrasound is used to detect abnormalities that lie deep in the glandular tissue or to confirm their benign nature by demonstrating cysts or thickened glandular tissue of normal texture. Mammograms of this type of breast are usually dense and therefore less informative.

Discrete masses

Ultrasound is highly reliable in differentiating solid masses from cysts; simple cysts do not require any further evaluation, although they may require decompression if symptomatic. Confirmation by aspiration is unnecessary and multiple punctures would have to be performed if they are multiple, as is very commonly the case. Fine needle aspiration cytology (FNAC) is indicated for all solid and indeterminate lesions because of the overlap of ultrasound features between benign and malignant masses. Although positive cytology is very reliable evidence of malignancy, cytology cannot exclude malignancy with certainty (mainly because of the possibility of a sampling miss) and the significance of a negative result must be evaluated in relation to the size of the mass (if large enough, there is less possibility of sampling error) and the nature of the specimen (a cellular sample is more reliable than scanty smears). Sampling errors can be improved by using ultrasound to monitor the position of the needle tip. Mammograms are often unhelpful in the diagnosis of lumps in younger women with dense glandular tissue which degrades the diagnostic value of X-rays. If these non-invasive (or, if FNAC is included, minimally invasive) examinations indicate that the lump is benign, it can safely be left in situ and the patient followed clinically.

For lumps that are suspicious on palpation, the ultrasound findings do not change the indications for surgery unless a definitely benign lesion that explains the suspicious palpable mass is revealed (e.g. a tense simple cyst which may be felt as a hard mass). For 'probably malignant' masses ultrasound is not indicated — the diagnosis must be confirmed by histology — though it can be useful to measure the size of the lesion, evaluate the extent of the disease and the status of the regional lymph node.

Other indications

Ultrasound is particularly helpful for masses in the augmented breast because the prosthesis does not interfere with the detectability of breast disease, a difficulty with X-ray mammography. In addition, silicone granulomas have a pathognomonic echogenic appearance on ultrasound and so can be reliably diagnosed. Ultrasound is valuable for monitoring mastitis because abscess formation that usually requires surgical drainage is readily detected[10]. Postoperative fluid collections are easily evaluated with ultrasound. Rarely, ultrasound demonstrates

Table 11.2	Indications for breast ultrasound	
General Indications	
Palpable abnormalities	
Benign or equivocal solitary mass	Cysts can be diagnosed reliably and needling avoided
Multiple masses	Solid lesions can be differentiated from cysts and biopsy directed appropriately
Mammographic abnormalities	
Non-palpable nodule	Solid lesions can be localised for needling or excision
Dense breasts or asymmetry	Occult and impalpable lesions can be detected
Special situations	
Inflammation	If cavities develop, percutaneous drainage may be indicated and is best guided by ultrasound
Tender breast	Ultrasound is better tolerated than mammography
Augmented breast	Ultrasound is unaffected by the prosthesis Silicone granulomas are easily diagnosed
Problems in pregnancy and young women	Ultrasound is free of radiation risk

that a clinically diagnosed breast tumour actually originates from an extramammary site, such as the pleural cavity or from the chest wall musculature.

Evaluation of mammographic abnormalities

As mammograms have become used more frequently, both for symptomatic women and for screening, the problem of evaluating indeterminate abnormalities has become more common. All mammographic abnormalities must be examined by careful palpation; lesions that were not felt initially may be located with the additional information provided by the mammogram. The management then is the same as other palpable abnormalities. If still impalpable, ultrasound is useful both for characterisation (is the lesion a cyst?) and for biopsy guidance.

Nodules

If nodules are demonstrated on the initial mammogram, ultrasound is indicated before additional X-rays are taken. About a quarter turn out to be simple cysts which do not require either additional views, aspiration or follow-up[11]. If the nodule is solid on ultrasound and it is new, excision biopsy is usually required because neither mammograms nor ultrasound can prove that it is benign. Solid lesions detected on the first screening mammograms pose a problem: even if the lesion is judged to be benign on careful evaluation of both the mammogram and the ultrasound, FNAC is needed (under ultrasound guidance if impalpable) because of the morphological overlap between benign lesions and some forms of breast carcinoma. Lesions that are benign on all these tests can be safely followed-up in the clinic.

A different problem arises when ultrasound fails to demonstrate a presumed cyst: since cysts are so obvious on ultrasound, failure to demonstrate the lesion means that it is not a simple cyst and the management then depends on the mammographic features. The majority of such lesions are benign (fibroadenomas, benign mammary change, or intramammary lymph nodes), but colloid carcinomas can be difficult to detect.

For impalpable lesions that are visualised on ultrasound, biopsy or preoperative localisation is better performed under ultrasound guidance as this is simpler for the patient and more precise than mammographic localisation. Naturally, mammography must be used for lesions that cannot be visualised on ultrasound.

Microcalcifications

As mentioned in previous chapters, the detection of microcalcifications outside a mass is very difficult on ultrasound. However, coarser, clumped calcifications can sometimes be demonstrated as bright echoes with or without shadowing, allowing the area to be aspirated or localised under ultrasound control. Microcalcifications may be accompanied by an abnormality of the surrounding tissue and this can often be detected on ultrasound.

Asymmetry

Asymmetry without a palpable abnormality is usually a normal variation. Ultrasound is indicated if there is suspicion of some other abnormality hidden within the mammographic density.

Stellate lesions

Stellate lesions may be due to breast carcinoma, benign breast change of the sclerosing type (i.e. sclerosing adenosis, radial scar) or to postoperative scars. Ultrasound may reveal a focal shadowing area and thus be useful for localisation but it is important to note that non-visualisation on ultrasound does not exclude an abnormality or indicate that the changes are definitely benign.

Screening

The goal of screening is to detect non-palpable carcinomas; palpable lesions should have been detected by self-examination and, anyway, are usually further advanced so that an impact on survival is less likely. Because ultrasound rarely detects non-palpable and X-ray negative carcinomas (none of 15 carcinomas[12], none of 587[13], one in 61[14]) and cannot detect microcalcifications, it should not be used alone for screening. It is generally held to be useful as part of a combination with mammography, though this has not been proven to be beneficial in reducing mortality or to be as cost-effective as mammography alone.

There are few reports on the use of ultrasound in screening and in these, now-obsolete static scanners were used[15,16]. Though the wide field of view they provide is a potential advantage for screening, the large number of images required to encompass the whole breast adds to the expense. In addition, dynamic and Doppler diagnostic criteria cannot be used with static scanners. Examining the whole breast with a real-time scanner and recording the images on a video tape recorder is another possible method. The most efficient way is for the scan to be performed by skilled sonographers but this is probably not cost-effective and quality of the examination is very difficult to control.

REFERENCES

1. E.A. Sickles, R.A. Filly, P.W. Callen: Breast cancer detection with sonography and mammography: comparison using state-of-the-art equipment. AJR 140; 843–845, 1982.
2. W. Schmidt, G. van Kaick, A Müller, et al: Ultrasonic diagnosis of malignant and benign human breast lesions. Ultrasound Med Biol 9 (suppl 2); 407–414, 1983.
3. R.L. Egan, K.L. Egan: Automated water-path full-breast sonography: correlation with histology of 176 solid lesions. AJR 143; 499–507, 1984.
4. D.B. Kopans, J.E. Meyer, K.K. Lindfors: Whole breast US imaging: four-year follow-up. Radiology, 157; 505–507, 1985.
5. J.A. Smallwood, P. Guyer, K. Dewbury et al: The accuracy of ultrasound in the diagnosis of breast disease. Ann R Coll Surg Engl 68; 19–22, 1986.
6. E. Tohno, E. Ueno, Y. Hirano, et al: Sonographic diagnosis of breast diseases: comparison with other diagnostic methods. Jap Jnl Med Ultrasonics 16 (suppl I); 493–494, 1986.
7. N. Hayashi, N. Tamaki, N. Yonekura et al: Real time sonography of palpable breast masses. Br J Radiol 58; 611–615, 1988.
8. P.A. van Dam, M.L.A. Van Goethem, E. Kerschot, et al: Palpable solid breast masses: retrospective single and multimodality evaluation of 201 lesions. Radiology 166; 435–439, 1988.
9. P.J. Dempsey: The importance of resolution in clinical application of breast sonography. Ultrasound Med Biol 14 (suppl 1); 43–48, 1988.
10. W.J. Leucht, D.R. Rabe, K. Humbert: Diagnostic value of different interpretative criteria in real-time sonography of the breast. Ultrasound Med Biol 14 (suppl 1); 59–73, 1988.
11. V.P. Jackson: The role of ultrasound in breast imaging. Radiology 177; 305–311, 1990.
12. S.A. Feig: The role of ultrasound in a breast imaging center. Semin Ultrasound CT MR 10; 90–105, 1989.
13. C. Kimme-Smith, L.W. Bassett, R.H. Gold: High frequency breast ultrasound. Hand-held versus automated units; examination for palpable mass versus screening. J Ultrasound Med 7; 77–81, 1988.
14. E.A. Sickles, R.A. Filly, P.W. Callen: Benign breast lesions: ultrasound detection and diagnosis. Radiology 151; 467–470, 1984.
15. L.W. Bassett, C. Kimme-Smith, L.K. Sutherland, et al: Automated and hand-held breast US: effect on patient management. Radiology 165; 103–108, 1987.
16. T. Wagai: Results of Screening trials in Japan. Ultrasonic Examination of the Breast, edited by J. Jellins and T. Kobayashi. John Wiley, 1983, pp 275–281.